"Dr Silvia Pfeiffer has an extensive background in computer science and healthcare consulting in a wide range of health environments, and as such is excellently qualified to write this book *Beyond the Clinic – transforming your practice with video consultations.*

Professor Peter Yellowlees, Past President, American Telemedicine Association.

"Dr Silvia Pfeiffer is passionate about enabling medical video consultations in Australia – her experience in this industry is quite unique."

Anita Mustac, Founder of online mental health service Dokotela, https://www.dokotela.com.au/

"Dr Silvia Pfeiffer has an amazing vision for what is possible in the technological side of telehealth, and pairs this with a genuine interest in the needs of health professionals. In the fast-moving world of digital health, early-movers like Dr Silvia Pfeiffer have a wealth of valuable insights to share."

Karen Finnin, Director of Online Physio, https://www.online.physio/

"Where healthcare meets technology, it is always hard to find someone who really understands the unique challenges that are present – Dr Silvia Pfeiffer gets it!"

Greg Borman, Director of online occupational therapy service Biosymm, http://www.biosymm.com/

BEYOND THE CLINIC

TRANSFORMING YOUR PRACTICE WITH VIDEO CONSULTATIONS

SILVIA PFEIFFER

Published in Australia by SJ Publishing

Postal: Parcel Collect 10010 41596, 12 West Parade,
West Ryde, NSW 2114, Australia.
Tel: +61 401 384 041
Email: info@sjpublishing.press
Website: www.sjpublishing.press

First published in Australia 2018
Copyright © Silvia Pfeiffer 2018

National Library of Australia Cataloguing in Publication entry

A catalogue record for this
book is available from the
NATIONAL LIBRARY OF AUSTRALIA — National Library of Australia

ISBN: 978-0-6483330-1-2 (paperback)
ISBN: 978-0-6483330-2-9 (epub)

Cover layout and design by Geopherae
Typesetting by Sophie White

Printed by Createspace

Disclaimer: All care has been taken in the preparation of the information herein, but no responsibility can be accepted by the publisher or author for any damages resulting from the misinterpretation of this work. All contact details given in this book were current at the time of publication, but are subject to change.

The advice given in this book is based on the experience of the individuals. Professionals should be consulted for individual problems. The author and publisher shall not be responsible for any person with regard to any loss or damage caused directly or indirectly by the information in this book.

This book is dedicated to clinicians, nurses and health-care professionals who work day-in day-out on improving patients' lives. It is to you that I bow, that I show all my respect, and that I'd like to offer my digital knowledge in an attempt to help you ease some of the burden you carry.

With deepest admiration,

– Silvia

ACKNOWLEDGEMENTS

*"Adaptability is key to survival in
the age of digital Darwinism"*
– Rob Gonda, Forbes Technology Council

I have a background in digital technology. I was part of turning the World Wide Web into what it is now. And yet, I find myself at times lost in the speed of change that digital technologies are inflicting on the world. Many people in my generation have given up trying to stay on top of change, trying to adapt to the new efficiencies that digital solutions can bring. The younger generations don't appreciate how much easier it is for them to be able to start from a blank piece of paper than to have to unlearn habits that used to be productive but are now just counter-productive. That is, until they get overtaken by the next generation that has just grown up with the next wave of digital technology.

Whenever I feel stuck, I reach out to people who understand the world around me better, understand the new rules of interaction, understand what digital solutions are the ones that will help take my efforts to the next level. I also reach out to people who are similarly stuck like myself and we figure out together how to move to the next level.

It is to you all, my friends, coaches, mentors, colleagues, partners and customers that I'd like to send a word of thanks. You know who you are, so let me just mention a few of you by name that have made a big difference in getting this book done.

Thanks to Andrew Griffiths, Glen Carlson, Sarah Wentworth-Perry, Sarah Bartholomeusz, Sonja Walker and many other friends of DENT for making me accountable, providing the tools and the encouragement to write the book.

Thanks to the team at iinspire media: my publisher Julie Postance, my editor Amanda Spedding, and my typesetter Sophie White. You've been efficient and responsive to all my needs and helped me navigate the complexities of putting a book in the market.

Thanks to Bill Simpson-Young, Terry Percival, Shelley Copsey, Adrian Turner, Phil Morle, and many other ex-colleagues at NICTA/CSIRO for providing the basis that allowed me to learn about telehealth and believing in my abilities to create a software system that can help clinicians make telehealth come alive.

Thanks to my co-founder Nathan Oehlman for sticking with me through all the time it took me to understand the needs of healthcare businesses that convert to telehealth and for turning these learnings into software.

Thanks to our current team at Coviu, including Jo Childs, Suzie Miller, Kaamraan Kamaal, Tom Quirk, June Brunken, Linzi Fine, and Anton Cush who have patiently awaited the finalisation of this book so it may function as a compass.

Thanks to Georgina Ibarra, Jeff Wang, Briely Marum, Pete Fields, Cathy Lill, Damon Oehlman, John Judge and many other ex-colleagues at NICTA/CSIRO who contributed to the original creation of Coviu while we were learning about the needs of healthcare businesses.

Thanks to Joanne Blackbourn, "Auntie" Lois Birk, Eileen Kalucy, Jenny Rayner, Julia Martinovich and the rest of the team at Royal Far West School where the idea for Coviu was born and my first experiences with telehealth were formed.

Thanks to Rebecca Sutherland, Greg Borman, Dale Bailey, Karen Finnin, Richard Harvey, Anita & Zelko Mustac, Carole Paterson, Costa Intzirlis, Rob Seiler, Wendy Phillpotts, Frankie Tait, Glen Smith, and many more of our customers who have all helped shape our understanding of telehealth.

And thanks to my amazingly talented son Benjamin Schaaf and my wonderful husband John Ferlito who are always happy to support me in my new endeavours that invariably lead to less family time. I love you both with all my heart and am humbled by the digital talent in our family.

CONTENTS

Section 3. Undertaking a transformation project ‎67

Section 4. We need to get everybody on board ‎95

Section 5. Getting technology fit for your workflows ‎123

FOREWORD

By Professor Peter Yellowlees, MBBS, MD
Past President, American Telemedicine Association.
Professor of Psychiatry, and Vice Chair for Faculty Development.
Department of Psychiatry, UC Davis
Author of *Telepsychiatry and health technologies
– a guide for mental health professionals*

Dr Silvia Pfeiffer has an extensive background in computer science and healthcare consulting in a wide range of health environments, and as such is excellently qualified to write this book, *Beyond the Clinic – transforming your practice with video consultations.*

The book has two main advantages over a number of other similar publications currently on the market. Firstly, it is very much a "how to" manual focusing primarily on the business implementation aspects of introducing video consultations into almost any type of health practice or clinic, and as such is full of sound advice gained through her practical experiences. Secondly, the book is an easy read, with many lists, key points and opportunities for readers to reflect on their own practice environment and personalise Dr Pfeiffer's advice and proposals.

Dr Pfeiffer herself, throughout the book, comes across as a visionary thinker with an eye always on patients and the provision of excellent care. She is someone who clearly sees the future and has written a book to help implement that future by changing healthcare systems into hybrid environments, where patients from many specialty areas are treated both online and in-person. She describes the many opportunities that there are to use video conferencing to improve the practice of medicine generally, and readers will have their eyes opened as they explore the range of case examples she cites.

I hope this book will be widely read and will assist many clinicians as they implement video conferencing in their practices, and congratulate Dr Pfeiffer on an excellent product.

PY July 2018.

INTRODUCTION

The purpose of this book is to provide you, the healthcare professional, with ideas for transforming your business for a digital future. It is a guide on how to successfully introduce video consultations into your healthcare business. The goal is to create more flexibility for your patients and clinicians but also make more money along the way and transform your business sustainably.

It is very clear that digital is going to substantially disrupt the way healthcare works, and telehealth is one substantial aspect of it. Telehealth projects have been run for many years and their clinical effectiveness has been proven. With the availability of bandwidth, affordable high-definition hardware and highly flexible, workflow-aware software, now is the time for telehealth to become a standard way of delivering healthcare.

With the ubiquity of mobile phones, consumer behaviour has changed towards all services in life. This change is not passing by healthcare and will substantially change how consumers look after their health and what they expect from their healthcare providers. Are you prepared for the change? Are you ready to embrace video consultations as a new delivery mechanism of services? Information about how to introduce video consultations is confusing. It often focuses on technology exclusively and doesn't consider the implications on operations or how to make the new service work financially.

As the founder of Coviu, a video consultations solution provider, I have worked with many healthcare businesses and seen many successful digital transformation projects, but also many projects that failed. I can provide realistic advice for practice owners on every aspect of the transformation process from idea through service design, training, pilot introduction, all the way to business-as-usual.

I've worked with not-for-profit organisations, specialist practices, GP clinics, Allied Health practices such as psychologists, physiotherapists, audiologists, dietitians, speech pathologists, exercise physiologists, and many more. I've worked with businesses that decided to go all-in on providing an online service exclusively, as well as with practices that decided to provide a hybrid online and in-person service. I'm passionate to share my experiences so we can all work together to innovate faster and more successfully in healthcare.

You might be curious to find out that my background is not originally in healthcare. I have a PhD in computer science from Mannheim University in Germany. I actually moved to Sydney, Australia, in 1999 to work for the Australian government research organisation CSIRO and invent new uses of digital media technologies. Later, I developed world-leading online video applications at Google, YouTube and Mozilla, and have co-authored standards in Web video technology at the W3C and published two text-books about HTML5 video.

In 2013, a project with a local school on telepractice brought me into the field of health consultations, which re-ignited my long-held passion to work in healthcare. My experiences in this project and several others that followed encouraged me to create the Coviu software and to write this book.

Healthcare businesses are busy, so it's difficult to experiment with innovative service models without disrupting an existing business. Often, a single clinician simply starts to experiment on their own schedule e.g. with Skype consultations, but then they hit problems such as how to transact payments, how to share medical imaging, what can be charged on Medicare, and how to integrate with the practice's appointment booking system. These problems are both technical (check out Coviu for a technical solution) and operational and suddenly everyone in the practice needs to get involved.

My goal with this book is to help you plan properly for an introduction of video consultations, get everyone on board, execute a successful pilot project and follow on to successfully transform your business.

How to read this book...

This book has been written as a step-by-step guide that you can follow along chapter by chapter as you plan and execute your introduction of a new video consultation service.

There is some duplication between different chapters, but that's because you will need to revisit challenges at different times.

Another reason for some duplication is that not everyone will read the book from front to back. The chapters have therefore been written so they can stand alone, and you can jump straight into a specific topic to get all the relevant information. This is particularly useful when you've worked through the process once and want to get back to a specific challenge selectively.

I'm available at **silvia@coviu.com** if you need further information or have any comments.

1

The time for video consultations has come

1

WHY PRACTICES NEED TO EMBRACE DIGITAL

Digital as an opportunity

The world is changing, and technology is all around us. I recently took a trip to Africa for safari and even there, where the native Masai continue to live their lives traditionally, I found that they own a mobile phone and are on the Internet. I was shocked to find wireless access in our tented camp out in the middle of the Serengeti.

All aspects of our lives are going digital – we share images and messages with friends on WhatsApp, we save documents in the cloud, and we do video calls with family or customers on Skype, Facetime or Google Hangouts. My son, who is in his early twenties barely sees his friends in-person. My husband works in a large corporate and has a great number of his meetings via video-conference. Yet, our medical practices still mostly deliver consultations as face-to-face sessions and some still do everything on paper. Healthcare is one of the last markets to embrace everything digital.

Now, since you're interested in video consultations, I'm going to assume you already have an interest in digital technology and your practice is probably using a practice management software. You might even have tried Skype and dabbled with the idea of setting up a new service for your patients to reach you via video online for health consultations.

There are many opportunities for healthcare businesses that embrace new technology. The advantages apply to your business, your clinicians and your patients. There is huge potential for growth of your business, since you can extend your services beyond the boundaries of your immediate neighbourhood and reach more patients. Your clinicians can adopt flexible working hours — possibly even offer out-of-hours services — from home and spend more time with the children. Patients can receive care when they need it wherever they are all while retaining continuity of care.

All of this applies to medical specialists and GPs as much as to Allied Health professionals. Many years of telehealth trials across different healthcare fields have resulted in studies that prove the clinical effectiveness of telehealth, particularly in mental health, emergency medicine, fields requiring ongoing therapy, family health, ophthalmology, dermatology and many other specialist fields.

Healthcare is changing

The way we deliver services in healthcare is not just changing because of the introduction of computers. Our modern healthcare systems were designed in an era where most illnesses were episodic – you'd go to the doctor or a specialist to "get fixed". However, the major current challenges our healthcare system faces are around chronic and complex health conditions which require ongoing efforts of prevention and management typically from a set of clinicians of multiple disciplines.

Around the world we are seeing healthcare systems trying out new models that include replacing the current fee-for-service model with value-based reimbursements or capitation-based payments. Where we will end up is as yet unclear, but change is certain.

Another factor that is changing healthcare is the increasing acknowledgement that the patient is at the centre of their own health and needs to be a responsible participant in keeping themselves healthy. The increasing introduction of mobile health apps and online information gives the patient the tools to look after themselves. Clinicians are embracing this by transitioning to patient-centric care – not just telling the patient what to do, but educating and empowering them in their decision making, giving them options, taking the personal situation into account, and coordinating more personalised care.

The introduction of precision medicine brings digital technology into the realm of patient-centric care. Precision medicine customises medical treatments or products for the individual patient based on their genetics or other molecular or cellular analysis. Digital technology has made it possible for us to subclass diseases into smaller patient populations where we better understand how to treat them successfully.

All of these changes in healthcare have something in common: they need more communication, collaboration and coordination between the patient and their clinicians as well as between the treating clinicians. Realistically, we can only satisfy the increased communication and data sharing needs through digital technology.

Embrace the change

You may like or hate technology, and you probably hate change, but it is far easier – and frankly more fun – to embrace the change and take advantage of it than to resist it and be left behind. Right now, you have the advantage of being at the forefront – you can make small changes at a time to ease your way into the new future. You can be the captain of change to your practice and contribute to the larger conversation. Wait too long and your practice will be forced to change to models that others have developed or become a dinosaur – just look at the DVD rental industry (Blockbuster, Video Ezy).

Video-consultations will soon be an integral part of providing a healthcare service by every professional. Most healthcare consultations don't require touch, so the hybrid model of holding in-person as well as online consultations makes the most sense.

A number of years from now that will change even further. Cheap consumer devices are starting to emerge for taking vital signs and pathology at home. Even implanted cardiac monitors can now be on the Internet. Finally imagine the use of a full-body haptic suit like the Teslasuit to provide virtual reality physiotherapy. These Internet-enabled consumer devices will in the not-too-distant future allow us to completely replace all needs for in-person health consultations. But let's stay with what is possible right now and start our transformation journey with simple video consultations.

QUICK EXERCISE

What has made you consider introducing video consultations? Take some notes and start considering what digital healthcare means to you?

2

VIDEO CONSULTATIONS ARE A TYPE OF TELEHEALTH

Terminology

This book is focusing on video consultations, which is part of the broader area of telehealth or telemedicine, which in turn are part of digital health.

The terminology in the digital healthcare space is still evolving, so I've chosen the specific term "video consultations" to signify the use of secure video connections by health professionals. This is roughly equivalent to the term "telemedicine" used in the USA to signify the use of telecommunication technology to provide clinical health care from the distance. In Australia, we often call this "telehealth".

"Telehealth", however, is also used for services that refer to the use of email, phone, or messaging to deliver clinician services, or remote monitoring devices. While these are not the focus of this book, they are still relevant even in a video consultation context: email, phone and messaging are often necessary communication components to prepare for a video consultation, and an ability to bring a remote health monitor into a video call can be advantageous for an online consultation.

"Digital health", in contrast, includes any use of new technologies to help address the health problems faced by patients. This may encompass:

- Mobile health data apps
- Consumer devices in health
- Remote monitoring devices
- Image or video-sharing services
- Patient portals
- Store-and-forward health services, such as via email or messaging
- Phone-based real-time health counselling
- Video-based real-time health services ("video consultations")

Don't let the terminology confuse you – we'll use "video consultations" and "telehealth" interchangeably in this book, but feel free to also use "telemedicine" or "digital health" if you feel more comfortable with these.

Application areas

Of all the different types of digital means of delivering health services, video consultations are the closest in results to seeing a clinician face-to-face. Telehealth, and video consultations specifically are used for cases as diverse as:

- Diagnostics
- Treatment
- Prevention of disease and injuries
- Research and evaluation
- Continuing education of healthcare providers
- Individual or group therapy
- Post-operative follow-ups
- Operations
- Care management
- Case collaboration
- Advice
- Monitoring

Essentially, all aspects of health service delivery can be supported and improved by using video consultations.

Users and locations

We already mentioned two of the key users of video consultations: clinicians and patients. But the people that are able to use video consultations is much more diverse than this. Telehealth, and video consultations specifically are used by people as diverse as:

- Patients
- Carers
- Nurses
- Pharmacists
- GPs

- Specialists
- Allied Health professionals

Interactions may be between people within the same group or between different groups, e.g. GP consulting with a specialist, or specialists consulting with each other.

As for where users may connect from, there is a vast flexibility in places. They can be as diverse as:

- Home
- Workplace
- National or international travels
- Shopping centres
- Sports centres/gymns
- Hotels
- Planes
- Community centres
- Schools
- Retirement homes
- Veteran organisations
- Non-for-profit health organisations
- Healthcare practices
- Hospitals
- Nurse stations

So there are many applications for video consultations across many different health services, users and locations. A lot of these will not be relevant to your specific business, but you should start thinking about the specifics of the service you'd like to offer.

QUICK EXERCISE

This chapter should have helped stimulate your imagination about what type of video consultation services you could offer. Write down a couple of ideas.

3

TELEHEALTH IS JUST HEALTHCARE DELIVERED VIA A DIFFERENT COMMUNICATION MEDIUM

Telehealth is not a medical specialisation

Working with several different organisations, I've seen whole divisions in hospitals being created as a new telehealth division. This was probably done for several reasons:

- **Financial:** the division was created as a new research project with its own funding.
- **Environment:** a controlled, separated environment is easier to keep interrupt-free and measure.
- **Technology:** expensive new hardware was required to install, including potentially specialised medical devices.
- **Administration:** the project introduced its own IT and management staff to deal with new administrative challenges.
- **Disruption:** a separate division meant no disruption to other departments.
- **Support:** technical support and user training could be provided in a separate area.

However, there are several downsides to such an approach, particularly since such a new division typically doesn't hire its own clinicians but makes itself available to other clinicians:

- How do you book a clinician's time between the telehealth department and their normal specialist department?
- To hold a video consultation, the clinician's office has to book a telehealth room and make sure to give the clinician enough buffer time to walk to the telehealth room and back.
- Make sure to prepare all the required digital and paper files for the consultations so the clinician can take them along to the consultation.
- How do you make sure the clinician can take notes in his normal EHR (electronic health records) system while being at another office where his setup is not available?

- How can the clinician get access to their collected health literature stored in their office while providing services from another office?
- How does the clinician's assistant find out when the clinician is ready with a telehealth consult while the clinician is in a telehealth office?

What is concerning about this approach is that health services don't change just because they are delivered over a different medium like video. The clinicians will continue to deliver the same service – the only difference is that it's online and not face-to-face.

If you introduce a telehealth department, you optimise for the wrong thing: you optimise for the administration and not for the clinical service. Such an approach will be counter-productive to converting video consultations into a standard service offering that is embraced by all clinicians.

Similar thinking also applies to smaller practices. Often, I have seen GP clinics or other practices create a specialised video consultation room. Reasons for doing this may be:

- **Administration:** admin personnel can set up the video call with a patient or another clinician while the clinician is still busy with other patients, so they can sort out any technology issues.
- **Technology:** specialised hardware was only necessary to be set up for one room.
- **Support:** Internet connectivity only had to be fixed up for one room.
- **Disruption:** since the clinician didn't need most of the other typical devices and practice facilities during the video call, this special telehealth room only needed a computer setup and could be a small "closet" room while another clinician could continue using a fully set up treatment room.
- **Environment:** the video consultation room could be away from the hustle of the clinic to provide a quiet environment.

Don't let yourself be tempted by these arguments – they lead you down the wrong path to a failed technology installation with no uptake because it's too much extra effort for the clinicians.

Business as usual needs integration

To embrace video consultations as a standard service in your business, you will want to encourage clinicians to provide healthcare services in the way they are used to, no matter whether it's an online or a face-to-face consultation. This is possible because the expense incurred for the technical setup is now minimal.

Every clinician's room needs a video consultation setup – regard it as just another tool that is part of your standard business setup like a telephone. With this in place, clinicians are enabled to make a simple decision on whether to see a patient via video or in person, because to them it's the same effort. It is not a special service with extra effort, but a choice based on what is more appropriate for a specific patient's situation.

The technical setup is not expensive these days; you simply need to buy a webcam, stick it on the clinician's computer and sign them up to a video consultation software. It's so simple, they will be able to manage the setup themselves.

Your goal as the business owner will be to introduce video consultations into clinicians' workflows as seamlessly as possible with as little disruption as possible. When a clinician gets to their next appointment in their scheduling software and can on-the-fly provide this either as a face-to-face or a video consultation, that's when you know it's all just healthcare and business as usual.

We'll talk later about the kinds of things you want to do with your software, hardware, and workflow setups to make this happen.

QUICK EXERCISE

Have you had any thoughts about how you would run video consultations in your business? Did you plan on dedicating specific time and a specific office to it? You can write down your current thoughts on how you think it can work and let's see this improve as you continue to work through the book.

4

TELEHEALTH REQUIRES MAKING CHANGES TO THE WAY YOUR BUSINESS OPERATES

It's about more than technology

Most books on video consultations or telehealth focus on the technology challenges that you will face, but very few discuss the changes that are necessary to the way your business operates. Don't think you can you just drop in some new software and it will magically turn your business into a successful digital business.

While basically everyone knows how to use Skype, creating a paid service based on video consultations is not as simple as adding Skype to your business. Even if you are a sole trader business and have full control over your workflows and computer setup – how are you going to share your medical documents, how do you do payments and reimbursements, what about consent forms, and how will you reach and market to patients?

Service design

Let's start with the biggest assumption: you are a key decision maker in your healthcare business and are able to introduce new service models. If not, then let's assume you've worked with a key decision maker and have their backing. Without top backing in your business, a digital transformation change like this is not going to be successful, so make sure you have the ear and support of the top decision makers before embarking on such a project.

One of the biggest changes you will have to make is to the work your staff and clinicians do – the processes and workflows they follow. Everyone in your business will need to be committed to making the change, otherwise you get competing opinions and diverging information about the new service. There may be a need for new job descriptions and staff training, so don't underestimate the effect on your people.

Think about any of the following issues and how you are going to address them in a hybrid in-person and online services business:

· Payments and reimbursements
· Appointment bookings
· Electronic health records
· Shared images
· Filling in of medical forms and consent forms
· Changes to working hours and introduction of remote work
· Software, hardware, network setup and quality
· Changes to your physical rooms and dress code
· Website setup and functionality
· Marketing to patients
· Tech support
· Regulatory issues

If you're planning on using video consultations as a booked service in a hybrid setup, you also need to make sure your practice is organised enough to stick to appointment bookings and the time they take; you don't want to have a patient wait online for a video call for more than a couple of minutes – by that time they might have walked away from their desk and got distracted with some other work. If you do run late, your practice staff will have to make sure to inform the patient.

As you can see, there's a lot to get organised. None of this is insurmountable though – you may even find a software solution that helps you integrate the new digital service into your existing service offering with minimal disruption. Then you need to focus on people issues and on getting word out.

A framework to help

The next sections of this book are going to help you through the process of preparing the new digital service in a way that addresses all the above issues step by step. I've developed a framework that we'll walk through so you can just work along. The framework brings together five vital aspects of successfully creating a new video consultation service:

· **Vision:** design the service you want to introduce.

- **Transformation project:** define a project that gives you a clear understanding of timelines and steps to undertake.
- **People:** define a communication plan that gets everyone on board.
- **Technology:** define the workflow and technology components of your service.
- **Sustainability:** build a profile for your service, promote it and get a reputation.
-

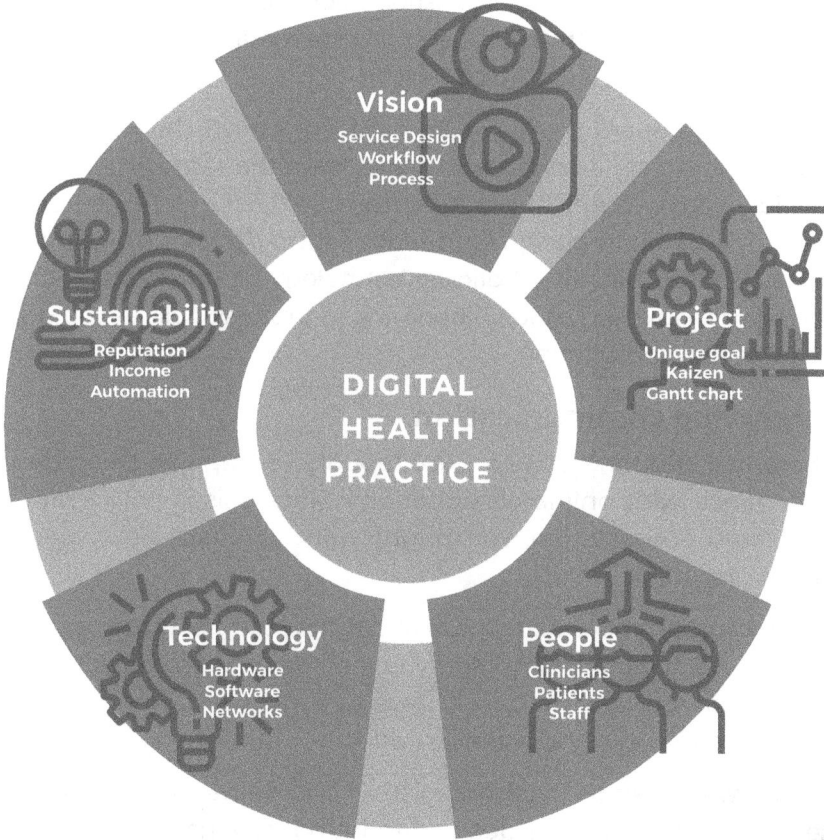

DIGITAL HEALTH PRACTICE

Vision
Service Design
Workflow
Process

Project
Unique goal
Kaizen
Gantt chart

People
Clinicians
Patients
Staff

Technology
Hardware
Software
Networks

Sustainability
Reputation
Income
Automation

QUICK EXERCISE

Have you had any thoughts about what your particular challenges may be, what changes you might need to make to your business? You can write down your current thoughts and we'll see how we can address them as you work through the book.

5

THERE'S NO CHANGE NECESSARY TO YOUR HEALTHCARE KNOWLEDGE

Telehealth is healthcare

Healthcare delivered online is no different from healthcare delivered via a digital interface such as video consultations. Clinicians still need their medical knowledge to question people about their issues, give advice, recommend treatment and provide therapy. Staff still need to communicate well with the patient.

The Medical Board of Australia's guidelines for technology-based consultation state essentially that they have the same expectations of high-quality medical practice from an online consultation as they do from an in-person consultation: **http://www.medicalboard. gov.au/Codes-Guidelines-Policies/Technology-based-consultation-guidelines.aspx** – so just keep behaving as professionally as you do in an in-person consultation.

Improving communication

There is something you can do, though, to improve the patient experience with online consultations. Since this is now a video-mediated conversation, you might want to adapt your style of communication.

Some clinicians have told stories about how they feel that being on video is like a performance and you feel like a TV presenter. There's some truth to that and you will develop some new communication skills as you become proficient on video.

I work with a speech pathologist who is delivering telepractice sessions to children. She decided to introduce a hand puppet into the session, which would say the things the children were meant to repeat. This made the speech pathology session feel more like a TV show for the children, but one where they were part of the show – an all-round success for everyone.

Some advice about things you can focus on:

- It's important you maintain eye contact with the patient as much as, or even more than you do in an in-person situation. You might be able to walk around and talk to them when they are in the same room – that will not work when on video (unless you have a camera that follows you around and you have a wireless microphone near your mouth).
- Ensure the patient is comfortable with the technology and the call at the beginning of the session – ask if they can clearly hear and see you and that they are in a quiet, private environment where they can focus on you.
- Speak slowly and clearly and if possible take notes in a shared whiteboard the patient can keep for later.
- Simply continue to follow your professional service standards, including taking notes about the consultation in your standard record-keeping software.

We've worked with many clinicians that were nervous about their first video call, but after a couple of calls got really used to it and soon found no big difference between delivering an online consultation and an in-person consultation. If you are very nervous, start with a mock call with a colleague or admin team member and pretend you're seeing a real patient with the whole process you would go through in a consult.

Suitability of video consultations

Not every patient visit is suitable for video consultations:

- Does the consultation require physical touch?
  If you know a physical examination will be required and there is no medical person near the remote patient who can "be your hands", you're better off deciding against a video consultation. If you discover a need for a physical examination during the call, schedule an in-person visit as a follow-up.
- Is the patient capable of getting the technology to work?
  It is best to have your practice staff do a test call with the patient before the actual consultation to confirm they can get the technology to work and that their bandwidth is sufficient. If a call between the patient and your practice staff doesn't succeed,

don't book a video consultation. Some software platforms have a self-test facility – you might be able to rely on that for confirming the patient is capable of getting a call going.

- Would the use of technology cause anxiety in a patient? This is particularly relevant in mental health patients. If the technology causes stress and anxiety, then it's counter-productive to the goals of the video consultation and the consultation should be taken in-person.

The latter two challenges are more pronounced with older patients. Problems will decrease over time as patients get used to the new technology and as your setup becomes increasingly standardised.

We have found that some patients really embrace the technology, while others loathe it:

- One study included an elderly lady who loved the video calls that she could take in her sitting room at home. She would dress up and put on makeup as if she were going out to see a doctor in person. She even prepared tea since for her it was a special event in her day and the clinician was a visitor to her home.
- In another study, an elderly man called up the help phone line before a video consultation and got increasingly agitated with frustration about problems he was having with the technology and eventually decided not to take the online call.

Clinicians and staff need to use their professional judgement with an understanding of the patients' lives and how the technology relates to the management of their health condition to decide if video consultations are right for a patient.

QUICK EXERCISE

If you have any ideas for communication techniques you want to try, feel free to write them down to keep a record of them.

6

YOU NEED A TRANSFORMATION PROJECT TO INTRODUCE VIDEO CONSULTATIONS

An adequate plan

We've talked about several of the challenges you will face when deciding to introduce video consultations. The best approach to making it a success to is to plan the introduction systematically. How much effort you put into the plan depends on the size of your project.

If you are a sole trading practitioner intending to give it a go for the first time, there's only a basic level of planning required. You still need to identify what you want to achieve and how you're going to decide whether your experiment was successful or not. You might want to test some assumptions:

- Test specific patient population's interest in video consultations.
- Test if you can reduce your rate of no-shows.
- Test usability of software by yourself and your patients.
- Learn about what functionalities you need in video consultations.
- Try to retain patients that are moving away or are travelling.
- Test if you can make money with a new care delivery model – this is what will ultimately make it sustainable.

Example project phases

Even in a small project such as this, you will need to go through certain phases and take notes along the way. Here's an example set of phases for a sole trading practitioner. Larger practices and clinics will need to add a lot more details.

Planning phase:
- Determine the goal of the project and have an initial long-term vision of where you may want to take this.
- Assess your technology environment – how ready for video consultations are you?
- Determine which software to use, and which criteria you might want to choose to pick a software.
- Make sure to be covered by insurance and regulatory aspects.
- Determine payments (or if you're just going to offer this for free for a trial project).
- Figure out reimbursement abilities for your patients.
- Determine what data to capture, e.g. patient feedback, rate of successful online consultations, issues encountered, benefits realised.

Setup phase:
- Acquire software, hardware and update network plans if necessary.
- Test the software, hardware and network setup with a couple of test calls.
- Recruit a couple of patients for test consultations and get them set up with software, hardware, network.
- Get patient consent to online consultations and data gathering.

Execution phase:
- Plan to run it for a couple of months to gather sufficient data.
- Hold consultations and gather data and learnings.
- It's best not to make any changes to your setup and processes during this phase, so you get clean data. If you have to, make sure to document the changes.

Assessment phase:
- It's important to have such a phase explicitly planned, so you can assess whether the project worked for you.
- Assess your notes and data taking any learnings and mid-project changes into account before you decide how to continue to introduce video consultations.

- Plan your next project, which may include a larger rollout, preparation of patient flyers, changes to your workflow, software integrations with your practice software and other EMR systems etc.

We're going to look into the details of what work goes into many of these phases in later chapters of this book. This is just to give you an initial idea of what you may need to consider in a transformation project. Don't be overwhelmed – take it one step at a time and things will fall into place.

QUICK EXERCISE

Consider the size of your project; keep it as small as possible but sufficiently large to give you an answer to at least one core question. What is the first core question you want to see answered?

7

PRINCIPLES WE FOLLOW IN THE BOOK: HYBRID CARE, MINIMAL DISRUPTION, SUSTAINABILITY

My goal: broad uptake

Telehealth and video consultations have been around for a while. But only recently times have changed and it is now possible to:

- Acquire consumer hardware (devices, cameras and microphones) that provide sufficiently high-quality video and audio calls to make excellent quality video calls.
- Get high enough quality standard Internet connections that provide sufficient bandwidth to deliver high quality video calls with little or no disruptions.
- Acquire user-friendly video consultation software at an affordable price that allows to develop a business model.
- Prescribe high-quality medical devices to consumers that can provide remote clinicians with the necessary medical data points and even pathology results to offer more than just advice over video calls.

Given this background, I believe it is now sensible to start a broad uptake of video consultations in healthcare by basically all professionals and clinicians.

Principles

Here are the principles that guide my advice in this book:

1. **Digital transformation:** video consultations are part of a transformation process the healthcare industry is undergoing, which is caused by technology and by a need to get exploding healthcare costs under control. As the healthcare industry is changing, so are care models, charging models, patient behaviour and, ultimately, clinician behaviour. It is a process that cannot be stopped, and it is best to embrace it early and in small steps.

2. **Continuous improvement (Kaizen):** digital transformation can seem daunting, but it can be taken in steps. We suggest defining

increasingly complex video consultation projects that embrace increasingly complex use cases. This is the most sensible way to embracing complexity, particularly in the face of a future that is unknown. And it will lead to the least necessary disruption to your existing business.

3. **Hybrid care:** in the past, it was the aim of video consultation projects to convert exclusively to an online service delivery model. While this is still a possibility, in this book we are mostly concerned with the hybrid-care case where some patients continue to be seen in person and others may be seen partly online and partly in-person. This is to maintain minimal disruption and lead digital transformation through Kaizen.

4. **Affordability:** we firmly believe that video consultations can be introduced through affordable technology and software without negatively impacting your existing business, so keep every step of the process affordable.

5. **Sustainability**: video consultation projects need to follow a clear goal of transforming a business in a way that ensures its long-term survival. Therefore, business models, charging models and reimbursements are a very important part to consider when setting up a new video consultation service.

QUICK EXERCISE

Write down what principles drive your video consultation project.

8

SHARING OUR EXPERIENCE FROM HELPING A DIVERSE SET OF PRACTICES IN AUSTRALIA

Video consultation services can take vastly different shapes. Here we introduce case studies of three very different businesses that have all made a difference to their clients. In the interest of transparency: all three are users of Coviu, **https://www.coviu.com**.

Case study 1: Physiotherapy – Greg Borman from *Biosymm,* https://www.biosymm.com.au

Biosymm is one of Australia's largest occupational physiotherapy providers specialising in early intervention injury management and ergonomic risk reductions. The company works with major retail, industrial, mining, rail and pharmaceutical clients, many of whom operate in isolated areas across Australia.

Greg Borman had a vision early on that would introduce video treatments to their corporate clients. He says: 'We have been performing telephone support for injured workers on mine sites since 2004. In 2014 we were part of a trial for a mining company to look at the benefits of video conferencing in the Pilbara. Although the outcome of the trial was successful, the technology was not user-friendly and the video quality was poor. In 2016 we began a pilot with a large chain of hardware stores where we again trialled videoconferencing and this time used a new program that is now helping us scale.'

Greg sees the opportunity that video-based triage and early intervention provide to reduce recovery times. There are many advantages to such an approach:

- Injured workers get assessed and treated almost immediately post injury ensuring they get the right advice in a timely manner – no matter where they are.
- Their supervisors get immediate advice as to whether a worker has to stop working or what types of efforts to avoid when they continue working.

- The employers save on lost time and workers' compensation injury claims.

Since implementing video consultations for their clients, *Biosymm* have achieved more than a 98% stay-at-work rate compared to an industry average between 40 and 60% (WorkCover Queensland Statistics 2015/16), which is consistent with their onsite physiotherapy co-located model.

Biosymm also provide physiotherapy to individual patients, so a mixed in-person and online service is provided. To make this work for their clinicians, *Biosymm* have integrated video consultation bookings into their practice management software. Availability is checked across all their clinicians throughout Australia and New Zealand. When a patient seeks to make a booking, the appointment is immediately scheduled right into the clinician's calendar. For the patients and employers, *Biosymm* have developed a branded mobile application that allows workers to join a video consultation through devices available at their workplace.

'One challenge is to get patients to embrace the new technology. We have introduced a telehealth concierge role which takes a person into the telehealth room just like a receptionist would greet them in a clinic. Once a patient experienced the consult, they see the value in the process and word of mouth would spread.'

The *Biosymm* service has been introduced in small steps with lots of measurement of impact along the say. Greg explains: 'When we were first looking, there was not much software out there that we could use because they had to provide a secure encrypted connection (we were dealing with medical information) to meet the Privacy Act restrictions. We then needed to get our team of physios on board with the idea that we could treat and manage cases via a video consult. This was no easy feat as physios are generally very hands-on in their treatment. But with some brainstorming and training we got them to believe it was possible and now the results speak for themselves.'

Case study 2: Speech pathology – Joanne Blackbourn from *SWAY,* http://sway.org.au

SWAY stands for "Sounds, Words, Aboriginal Language and Yarning" and is an oral language and early-literacy programme based on local Aboriginal knowledge, culture and stories. *SWAY* builds the capacity of rural and remote teaching staff through quality professional development and ongoing mentoring. *SWAY* is delivered by experienced speech pathologists, Aboriginal educators and teachers at the Royal Far West School in Manly, NSW.

Joanne Blackbourn, the leading speech pathologist of the *SWAY* programme says: 'SWAY is a classroom and targeted intervention programme that aims to improve the oral language and literacy outcomes of preschool and kindergarten students. The *SWAY* team travels out to rural and remote schools to provide onsite teacher training. During the course of the following year, the teaching staff receive mentoring via the Coviu video platform. The teaching staff benefit greatly from the support they receive through these ongoing remote mentoring sessions.'

The programme started with individual speech pathology telepractice sessions for individual children. The service delivery model has since evolved to small group speech pathology intervention that reinforces the learning objectives of the whole class programme. 'Working with rural and remote schools and preschools, we really needed a video platform that would be user-friendly, reliable, interactive and engaging for young children. High-quality audio and video using low bandwidth was also essential.' At that time, existing video conferencing platforms did not provide the functionality required. We worked closely with a research organisation to co-develop and trial a video platform. These features are now part of Coviu.

SWAY has developed into a fee-for-service programme. The *SWAY* team currently delivers remote speech pathology intervention and mentoring to six sites within NSW. Within the past three years, the *SWAY* programme has provided professional development training and mentoring to over 44 rural and remote teaching staff. Over 300 children have received targeted speech pathology interventions. 'Accessing speech pathology in rural and remote areas is tough. Families report having to travel many hours to attend appointments in regional centres. Research suggests that on average rural and remote children arrive at schools with language skills 18 months behind their metro peers. Without SWAY, many of these children would not have been able to receive the support they needed.'

Growing research supports the efficacy of speech pathology intervention and mentoring delivered via tele-practice. Our teams' vision is for all rural and remote communities to have equivalent access to speech pathology intervention, quality professional development and mentoring, as metropolitan areas.

Case study 3: Psychiatry – Anita Mustac from *Dokotela,* https://www.dokotela.com.au

Dokotela is an online provider of specialist mental health care consultations. A dozen highly-experienced psychiatrists, psychologists and paediatricians offer their advice on matters related to mental health via video calls online.

Mental health is a particularly interesting area to offer online advice for several reasons.

Seeing a psychiatrist about a mental illness often causes a negative stigma – patients may be treated as different, as if they are somehow less than other people. This is particularly true in rural and remote areas where it's almost impossible to hide that you are seeking help. Visiting a mental health specialist online is therefore often preferred by patients because of privacy issues.

In addition, the use of online consultations provides patients in rural and remote areas with access to specialists sooner and without the time and expense involved in travelling to major cities.

Finally, patients with severe mental health issues often find it difficult to leave their homes and face the world outside. Without the option of video consultations from home, these patients are likely to go untreated. Online consultations can get them advice earlier and more frequently.

The *Dokotela* service started with Skype-based mental health consultations by one psychiatrist, who was referred only via word-of-mouth of GPs. As the psychiatrist moved across the country and had to close down his brick-and-mortar business, he decided to move the private practice to an online service exclusively (he still works part-time at a private hospital).

He partnered with an experienced investment professional and together they set up a website. The website includes an online appointment booking facility, online payment functionality, and is using online video consultation rooms with built-in waiting room functionality. Increasing patient demand required extending the set of consultants. As they grew their business, they also hired a telehealth coordinator for patient support and to assist the specialists to ensure their practices run smoothly.

Anita says: 'Psychiatry is ideally suited to video conferencing. However, there are many logistical, administrative and technology hurdles that can quickly become overwhelming for the Specialist, GP, GP clinic staff and patient without the right technology and team in place to support the process.'

The *Dokotela* service is GP-referred, and the consultations are usually held in dual-care consultation where the patient joins the video consultation with their GP. Medicare rebates apply where the patient is situated in a rural or remote area as defined under the Australian Standard Geographical Classification and is more than 15km away from the consultant psychiatrist.

Anita is excited about the service's impact: 'The benefits for patients are very significant. It is timely (appointments within 48 hours), cost effective (due to the higher Medicare rebates available) and convenient for the patient. The collaboration between GP and patient facilitates a patient-centric collaborative approach.'

Scientific research has confirmed that it is possible for a clinician to build trust with a patient online, which is a core requirement for successful health outcomes, particularly in mental health.

QUICK EXERCISE

Write down any thoughts you have about the status of your business and what a case study about your business might look like after a successful introduction of video consultations.

CHECKLIST: ARE YOU READY TO MAKE A DIFFERENCE WITH VIDEO CONSULTATIONS?

Re-consider some of the key points discussed in this section:

1. Are you getting excited about the prospects of bringing change to your business?
2. What advantages do you want to give your clients/patients?
3. What opportunities do you want to bring to your business?
4. Are you ready to prepare a transformation plan and execute it?
5. Are you and your business ready to embrace new technology?

2

Imagine your future with video consultations

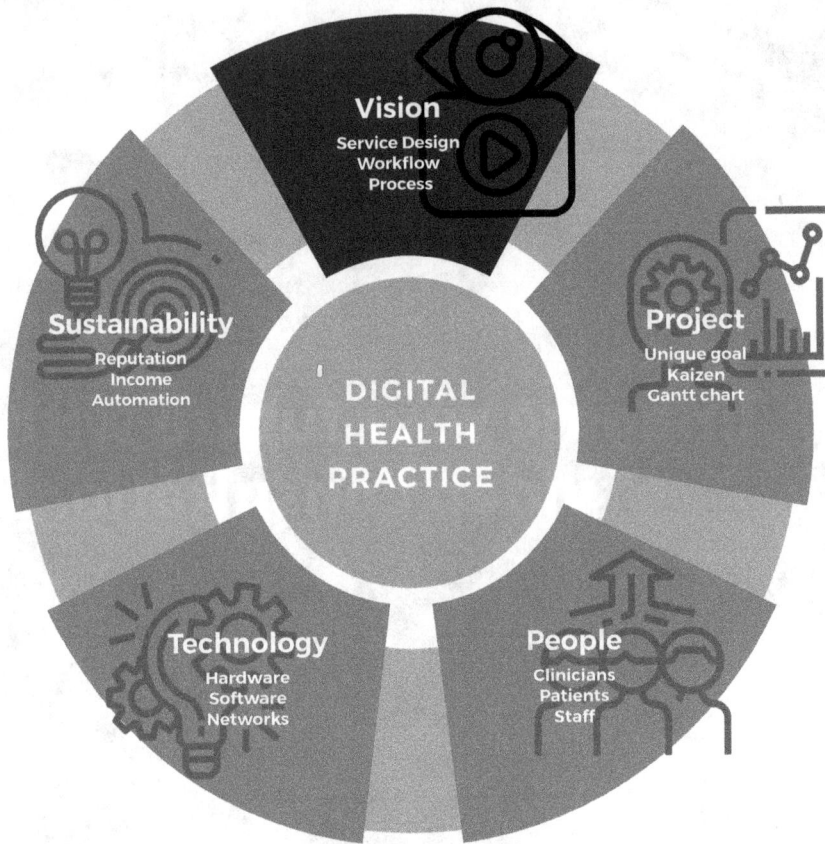

Vision
Service Design
Workflow
Process

Project
Unique goal
Kaizen
Gantt chart

Sustainability
Reputation
Income
Automation

DIGITAL
HEALTH
PRACTICE

Technology
Hardware
Software
Networks

People
Clinicians
Patients
Staff

VISION

In this section we're looking at the first component of the digital health transformation method: building a vision.

9

START BY IMAGINING WHAT THE FUTURE OF YOUR BUSINESS SHOULD LOOK LIKE

Think big

You cannot achieve a different future successfully without imagining it. So that's where we're going to start: with a big vision for your business. At this stage, think big and don't let yourself be limited by what you can afford or the first steps you're going to take. Dream! Just be a bit careful what you dream up – it might come true. ☺

As a clinician, you may decide to use video consultations as a retirement step to start cutting down on your work and help your existing patients from home. I've seen a number of psychiatrists close their physical practice and run a virtual practice completely from home. Alternatively, I've also seen the opposite: an occupational health business used video consultations to expand their reach across Australia and New Zealand and open new locations to cover a vaster range of time zones for in-person and video consultations.

If you had all the technology in the world that you can imagine and all the money in the world, what would your healthcare business look like? Maybe think back to when you started working in healthcare and what motivated you then. Did you want to eradicate a specific illness? Help a certain patient population? Be the best practice in the world? Or maybe simply reach the most difficult cases in your specialisation? Well, you know what? With the help of technology, there's never been a better time to make your vision come true than right now with the help of technology.

Let's brainstorm

What would you do if your practice wasn't limited by walls? If you could offer your knowledge, advice, therapy approach or insights to anyone in need anywhere?

Focus around a future where video consultations are a standard part of your digital practice. There may be more technology and changes necessary than just video consultations, but don't limit your thinking for now.

Make this about patients: who are you passionate to help? Who would you reach if you could? Would you specialise more on specific patient challenges or generalise more?

Make this about business: what would your practice look like? Would you grow and hire more clinicians? Maybe across more disciplines to offer more holistic health services to patients/clients? Would you open more locations to cover more time zones and larger regions? Would you offer out-of-hours services online?

Make this about clinicians: would you talk about more flexible working hours? Would you allow some from-home working time? Would you balance clinic hours and private consultations differently?

Make this about staff: what technologies would you have that simplify workflows and staff work? What extra staff do you need? What occupations do you require less of?

Make this about partnerships with other healthcare businesses: who would you collaborate with? Would you partner with other private practices, or maybe even with hospitals?

For the purposes of this book, we'll focus on the video consultation part of your vision as a core motivation to change, so let your imagination be carried by the possibilities of unlimited reach. You will notice that introducing the kind of flexibilities that video consultations allow has a vast impact on many aspects of your healthcare business.

QUICK EXERCISE

Write down some cornerstones of a vision for how your business will look after embracing video consultations and digital health.

10

WHAT POTENTIAL BENEFITS CAN YOU ACHIEVE FROM VIDEO CONSULTATIONS?

The benefits

Now that you have some ideas about where this may lead you, it's time to think about the benefits this can bring to all involved. This will help you prepare reasons to get everyone on board and help in bringing about behavioural change in colleagues and patients.

Here are some ideas of benefits that may motivate your clinicians, patients, and the business.

Advantages for clinicians:

· Ability to work from multiple locations, including when travelling.

· Ability for work-time flexibility, e.g. out of hours services.

· Ability to fit in consultations at short notice, e.g. when not at the office.

· Encourages holding more consultations by sticking to time limits.

· Ability to interact with distributed care teams/multi-disciplinary teams (MDTs).

· Encourages patients to engage more frequently and be more compliant.

· Ability to phase out of active work in a practice as a transition to retirement.

· Ability to start a practice without investment in brick and mortar.

Advantages for patients:

· Avoid travelling, particularly for emergencies and repeated therapy sessions – think about all the families and elderly citizens that are finding a trip to your practice a real burden.

· Get better service even if you live in rural or remote areas.

· Easier to fit in a busy lifestyle – convenience.

· Less risky for patients with mobility issues.

· No risk to pick up infections.

· Encourages quicker actions on health issues.

- More anonymity, particularly in mental health.
- Access to medical expertise that is not available locally/access to the best expert.
- Ability to have a carer join a consultation even if the carer can't spare the travel time.

Advantages for practices:

- Ability to extend practice-reach beyond the immediate neighbourhood.
- Ability to allow clinicians more flexible work hours and locations.
- Multi-location practices can more easily balance availability between locations.
- Ability to hire more clinicians for services without renting more space.
- Ability to diversify practice with several disciplines to provide a more inclusive and holistic health service to patients/clients while hiring more specialised clinicians.
- Ability to sell work-health services more cheaply and consistently to corporates.
- Ability for partnerships between specialist and GP practices to introduce dual-care services.
- Reduced no-shows with ability to convert patient to online consultations (reference: http://onlinelibrary.wiley.com/doi/10.1002/pdi.2078/abstract).

QUICK EXERCISE

There are many potential advantages with video consultations. Hopefully this has given you some ideas as to how it could help your business specifically. You can write down a couple of ideas.

11

WHAT DO YOU PERSONALLY WANT TO ACHIEVE? IMAGINE THE FUTURE FOR YOURSELF

Your personal why

Let's be selfish for a moment. Consider your role in the vision of your future digital healthcare business and have a think about what this might mean to you personally.

- What will your role be in a video consultation-enabled digital healthcare business?
- What do you hate about your current job and how can you make it better in your imagined future?
- What might a typical day at work in the future imagined business look like?
- What impact will the change have on your private life, your family?
- How will your interactions with patients look?
- Will you be spending less time in traffic and other stressful situations? What effect might all this have on your lifestyle?

If you're a clinician:

- What might a typical consultation look like? Imagine the kind of things you're doing in consultations right now and how you might be able to replicate them online. Always assume technology could make anything possible, including remote examinations.
- What might a patient's interaction with you look like, beginning at the moment they decide to contact you?
- Will your relationship to patients change? If you think it might suffer from not being face-to-face, what could you do to improve it?
- What will your interactions with other healthcare professionals look like, inside and outside your business?

- Will you be able to rearrange your days to, for example, spend more time with your children and maybe work in the evening, weekend or at night from home?

Thinking about the direct impact on your life and the improvements you can gain will make the vision much more real for you.

Your special requirements

As you analyse your future work interactions, you'll probably notice something interesting: you'll find that you have technology requirements that go beyond the capabilities of mere video conferencing software. There are workflows around appointment bookings and appointment reminders and waiting rooms and patient consent and data entry and of course payments and reimbursements that differentiate a video consultation from a mere video call with friends and are also substantially different from a corporate video conferencing call.

You might even consider the kind of interactions a clinician has with a patient during a consultation which might include scribbling notes on a pad, sharing flyers, forms or other documents, looking at medical imaging together, or writing prescriptions. These kinds of interactions are clearly not possible in standard video conferencing software. It's good to understand the limitations of video conferencing software because such software is often used to introduce video consultations. What you get by using such software is a restriction in the kind of video consultations you can hold. It's probably ok to start with (which is why many people have their first go at video consultations using Skype), but it's not sufficient when you try to scale it and make it a standard service offer. Consider specialised solutions like Coviu or Doxy.me or eVisit.

QUICK EXERCISE

Hopefully this has given you a better understanding of what you hope to achieve for yourself. You can write down a couple of ideas.

12

DON'T PLAN IN ISOLATION
- VALIDATE YOUR VISION WITH OTHERS

Extending your vision

It's very tempting to have a vision and not share it with others. Maybe you're a little embarrassed that you've not thought through all the details of how it might work and what everyone's roles are, so you're afraid to get questions you cannot answer. Don't worry about it. At this stage, you cannot know everything.

In fact, as part of defining your vision further, you need to interact with others. You need to get their opinions and insights and ideas to further develop your vision and validate your assumptions. Talk with everyone who may play a role in the future version of your business. Include other clinicians, practice staff, and specifically patients to see how they react. Maybe even talk to private health insurances about whether they'd support it. Work your industry network – even your professional association – to get feedback on your ideas.

Talk to patients

This is a good time to actually gather some information from your patients. Find out whether they would be keen to pick up such a service and recruit them as alpha testers. Ask what their problems are, whether they would be tech savvy enough to do a video call, what kinds of health services they would like to receive via video and talk about payments. Maybe do some brainstorming first so you can suggest a couple of services and see what they say about them. Find out if they'd be willing to pay privately for it, since this would be the easiest way. Some of the services your patients are after may actually have Medicare support, such as mental health sessions, so those are good to mention also.

Talk to staff

Talk with your practice staff about the idea. Find out what (if any) objections they have – they are the ones managing the appointments, payments and administrative processes around your business, so they need to be on board with this change. Don't ignore their concerns, but rather write them down so you can use this information to later discuss with a solution provider. Your staff might also know specific patients that would be useful as alpha testers, so get them to help and include them early – that will stop any resistance at a later stage.

Talk to other businesses

Make sure to use your professional network to talk to other practices that may have such a service running successfully – or those that have failed at setting it up beforehand. Learn from their lessons to avoid making the same mistakes. Talk to your industry body to find out where they stand and if they have any procedures or recommendations for telehealth. They may also have good information about regulatory, privacy, and reimbursement aspects.

Do some research

You can also conduct research in the scientific literature. Collect some articles and research publications about telehealth in your specialisation. They will give you an idea about what works and what doesn't work. However, take these publications with a grain of salt; they may be older and undertaken with complicated software or poor network connectivity. Keep a critical eye on the setup of the research projects and understand what might have led to success and what to failure. These articles are a great source from which learn.

QUICK EXERCISE

Make a list of some of the people and organisations you want to talk to and the research you want to undertake to develop your vision and understanding further.

13

WHERE THINGS GO WRONG: START WITH ONLY ONE SERVICE AND ITS VIABILITY

Focus, focus, focus

Now that you've developed a big vision about how the future of your business might look and have collected a lot of ideas about all the things you could do, it's time to return to reality. I'm pretty sure you've got a million ideas and are by now confused as to where to start. Let me confirm what you already know: the big vision cannot be achieved in one big step. We have to break it down.

In fact, I recommend introducing only a single service into your practice. And I further suggest doing it with a small trial – a small number of clinicians and a small number of patients for a fixed duration. This simplifies everything: it gives you more control of the transformation process, a simple technology setup, provides insights into your workflows, and allows you to expose and fix issues.

Even if you are doing this for a second or third project, it is still important to focus on a single extra service and to introduce your new services successively, otherwise you're taking on too much at a time and it will disrupt your existing business.

How to choose

So how do you pick your first service? That completely depends on your practice.

What are some of the **key challenges** of your practice? I'm going to list some examples that I've heard before, but you will need to find what is relevant to you.

- Maybe the key challenge of your business is that there are too many gaps in clinician schedules that you need to fill, so you need to reach more patients.
- Or your clinicians are all booked out, but many of your patients don't show up for their sessions.
- Maybe you can see that your patients' health is continuing to slip

despite them seeing you regularly and you want to introduce a different kind of service that includes a regular video check-up.

- Are you a specialist clinician who has been serving the bush through fly-in-fly-out (FIFO) but want to reduce your travelling while continuing to provide services where they are needed?
- Are you a family GP clinic and can see the challenges early-morning child illnesses pose on families and want to offer early-morning video consultations as a way for them to save time and hassle?
- Maybe you have just finished your medical studies and are considering opening a practice, but want to build in video consultations from the start.
- Are you a not-for-profit organisation who wants to help their members with counselling on a certain topic or even regular therapy sessions, but your members are distributed across the whole country?

Think about what in your current situation and business video consultations can improve.

Since we want to make this **financially viable**, can you create a first service directed by what can be reimbursed? Are there services that Medicare reimburses? Do you know if your patients will be happy with private payments? Can you find a corporate sponsor for an online service? Can you get any grants for doing such a project? Think creatively and discuss with your staff and patients and you will come up with a workable business model.

Can you choose a first service by looking at where there is **specific energy in your business**? For example, do your clinicians have a specialisation that could be a focus? Or is there a specific clinician who is particularly keen to be involved, or a specific staff member who is very supportive? Build on your business' strengths.

You can also choose your first service by **analysing your patients**. What do they specifically need? Do you have corporate clients, families, busy professionals, retirees? Each one of them has a different need and your focus should be on just one to make this work.

Finally, you should consider how **easy it is to take the service that you choose online**. Are there lots of paper materials involved in delivering the service, e.g. forms, flyers, assessment materials etc.? Can you get them digitised easily? Do you need specific medical devices to deliver the service or is a mobile phone's capability sufficient?

Advantages of uniformity

Try to set up a single uniform service first instead of doing random sessions for all kinds of services and patients. The advantages of making it uniform are manifold:

· Easier to market it to patients with a single flyer and marketing campaign.

· Easier to target it at one patient population with uniform needs and concerns.

· Easier to train your staff.

· Easier to prepare usable digital material during the consult.

· Easier to prepare successful workflows.

· If medical devices are required, you'll only need to buy one type and can distribute it to all your patients or partner practices.

· Easier to measure success.

With new service introductions you cannot make it simple enough – the more complexity you take out, the more successful your first transformation step will be.

This step is vital, so spend a lot of time thinking about what can work for your practice. If you do this right, your first video consultation service will get everyone on board, including your patients and staff. Your medical colleagues will look towards you, and you can be a part of successfully transforming the healthcare industry to the digital future.

QUICK EXERCISE

Use your gut feeling: what do you think should be the first service you offer online? Start exploring why you came up with that service, and jot down some notes about your intuition.

14

ADD DETAILS TO YOUR VISION: WORKFLOWS, PEOPLE ROLES, SYSTEMS, MONEY FLOWS

Meat on the bone

We're now focusing on the one service that you picked for your transformation project. Let's sketch out as many details about it as you can.

There are so many different use cases for video consultations that the details of the service you are setting up will be specific to you personally and to your business. Do consider the following issues:

Consultation

- Imagine a consultation and how it might differ from an in-person consultation.
- How would the work of the clinicians change?

Marketing

- How might a patient find out about the service? Would you have flyers in your existing practice? A digital newsletter? Articles on social media? Work with an insurance company to introduce the service?
- Can you get it listed somewhere where patients are looking for clinicians? Maybe an online directory?

Workflow

- How would a patient join the service? A common approach is: go to your website, book a consult online, receive an email, pay for the consult and join a call. But your service may need specific features – what are they?
- What might the work of your staff members look like? What new services would they need to provide? Think about having test calls with patients or other clinicians.
- What people do you think you need to hire to deliver that service?

Financial sustainability

· Who could be paying for the service? Is it the patient? Family and friends? The insurance? Medicare? An employer? Donations? Sponsorship? A government grant?

Technology

· You can also consider what software systems you might need, but it's a bit too early to worry about the solution. First, you need clarity on your service. You can always discuss your needs with a software provider at a later stage.

As you start thinking about these issues, discuss them with the people around you. Earlier we talked about sharing your big vision to get their input. Now it's time to get input on this specific service and the specific impact it might have on everyone.

QUICK EXERCISE

Consider the challenges that the introduction of this new service poses on clinicians, staff, and patients. You can take some notes.

15

WRITE DOWN YOUR VISION AND ADD USER STORIES

Project notes

You've brainstormed a lot of ideas in the previous chapters and you might even have started writing down some of these ideas about your big vision and the specific service you decided to focus on first. None of this needs to be complete yet, but the more you write down, the more concrete your service becomes.

If you haven't started a project book, now is a good time to begin. It's best to put all your thoughts in one place and continue to iterate there. This could also be a digital document you continue to improve. Create some sections and add to them as you learn more about your project. Some sections could be labelled "Overall Vision" and "First Project". Aggregate the notes you've taken while reading this book.

User stories

Next, we'll get some life into these ideas by creating user stories.

Make a section on "Clinicians" and what the daily life of a clinician looks like once your new service is introduced. Start with them getting up and end with them going to bed – what might happen in between? Where will they be when they will be seeing patients? In hospital, hospice, practice, at home, etc? If your practice is multi-disciplinary, consider each specialisation separately. How do they work together? Things become concrete when you're thinking them through with this much detail.

Similarly, make a section on "Patients" and consider what their interactions with a clinician look like. Start by describing their age, gender, profession and type of condition. You might need several example patients to cover your target population. Think through what touch points they might have with your practice and your clinicians. You can even find some photos online and put them next to your patient profiles and stories of how they would use the technology to make it more real.

You might also need a "Family member" user story. Particularly with small children, elderly patients or cognitively-disabled patients – interactions are often not just with a patient but also with a carer or family member. If your first project includes such types of patients, you'll likely need to think about what options for interaction with the clinicians the family member or carer may be able to get.

Create another section on "Staff" and consider the different staff members that may be affected. This may include your receptionist, potentially a video consultation coordinator, your IT support, your admin person and any other staff member. Write a user story about how their day looks and their involvement with the telehealth case for each one of them. Think about a standard day where everything works out and then about a miserable day where things go wrong.

User experience

This exercise is actually very good to start defining your user experience and workflows. Take your time – this may take a couple of days to put together. Leave enough space between the sections so you can enter more ideas at a later stage. This will be very useful for your conversations with your technology provider, because you will have plenty of questions to ask about the types of functionalities and user interactions you need.

QUICK EXERCISE

Are there any other users of your system that we've overlooked? You can take some notes here, but mostly, your project book should now keep your thoughts.

16

OPTIMISE YOUR VISION FOR PATIENT DESIRABILITY AND BUSINESS VIABILITY

Measure success

The first telehealth project that you're working on will need to satisfy a couple of requirements to be successful. You will want to measure your success, both quantitatively and qualitatively.

Start thinking about these goals now. Two of the most important goals in your service design will be that the service is desirable by patients and that a business model around it is viable. But there may be many more goals to optimise your project plan.

Define metrics

You can measure goals such as these quantitatively and qualitatively:

- **Staff buy-in:** e.g. 100% of staff had no problem with the new workflow and service; 'We found it easy to manage the old and new service workflows'.
- **Clinician acceptance:** e.g. all clinicians held video consultations – the goal of a minimum of 100 per clinician was successfully achieved.
- **Patient desirability:** e.g. 90% of patients had no problem connecting remotely; 'I am so happy about this service – I wouldn't have received the care I needed without it'.
- **Technology works:** e.g. 95% of scheduled calls took place, the rest were either no-shows or excessive firewalls or bandwidth-related failures.
- **Financially viable:** e.g. the consults were charged at $10 less than in-person consults but reduced our no-show rate by 90%; we therefore made more money from these than if they had been regular in-person consults.

Capture data

You will need to design into your project a way to capture the data, so it's good to start early thinking about what you might regard as success and what data you might want to capture to measure that success.

Poor metric results

Don't get discouraged if your metrics are poor at first. Poor results are an opportunity to improve. Maybe you don't need all your clinicians to hold video consultations. If you start with a couple of clinicians and some of them love it and others hate it, you learn something as well. Find out why they hate it, address their issues and improve the service. In fact, your goal might have been wrong – 100% clinician acceptance might be too strong a goal to push for. Set yourself realistic goals – maybe 20% is a good start and the rest is about discovering ways to improve.

QUICK EXERCISE

Add a "Success" section to your project book and write down your initial thoughts about what you regard as project success and how you'd like to measure it quantitatively and qualitatively?

CHECKLIST: DO YOU HAVE A VISION OF RUNNING YOUR BUSINESS WITH VIDEO CONSULTATIONS?

Re-consider some of the key points discussed in this section:

1. Have you started writing your plans down in a project book?

2. Have you formulated your overall vision and what benefits you can see in it for yourself, your practice, your staff, clinicians and patients?

3. Have you formulated your project focus and does this project include a single service only? Does it include workflows, people roles, systems, and money flows?

4. Have you spoken with your peers, staff, clinicians, patients and others about your ideas and validated some of your assumptions?

5. Have you started writing down what quantitative and qualitative goals you might want to achieve in this initial project?

3

Undertaking a transformation project

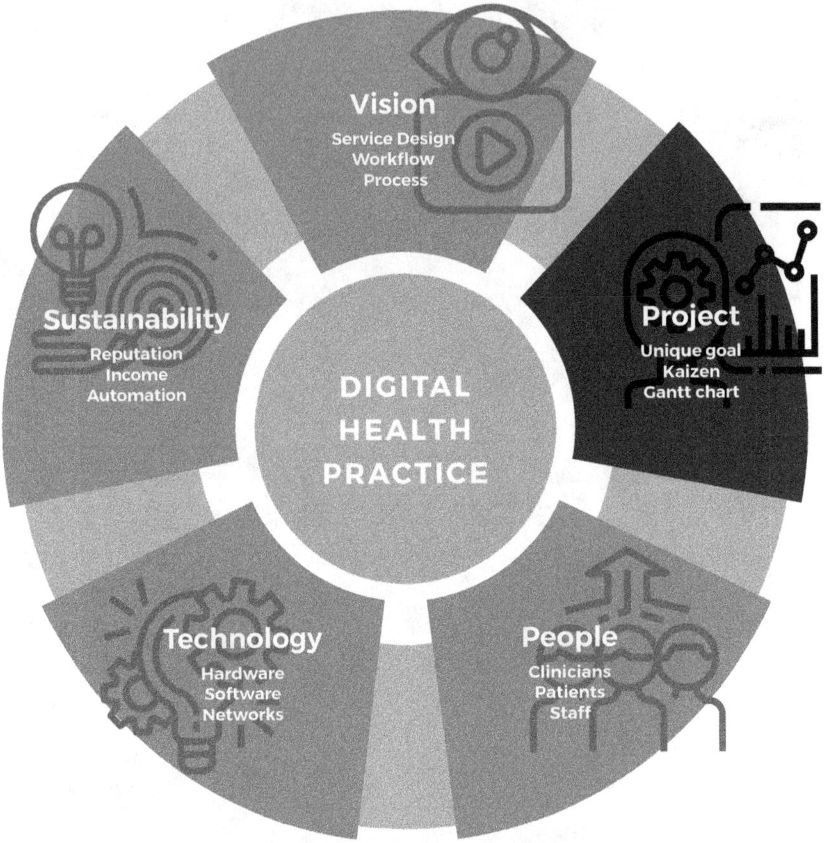
Vision
Service Design
Workflow
Process
Project
Unique goal
Kaizen
Gantt chart
People
Clinicians
Patients
Staff
Technology
Hardware
Software
Networks
Sustainability
Reputation
Income
Automation
DIGITAL
HEALTH
PRACTICE

TRANSFORMATION PROJECT

In this section we're looking at the second component of the digital health transformation method: project planning.

17

ADVANTAGES AND DISADVANTAGES OF DOING A PILOT PROJECT FIRST

Realising your vision

In the previous section you've outlined the first service that you will launch as a video consultation service. Now it's time to plan the steps towards the launch and put together a transformation project plan.

The first thing you might want to consider is whether you want to do a small pilot project to gather some experience before doing the proper project that leads to a sustainable service.

Pilot project

A pilot project is a small experiment that you can run with a single clinician and a hand full of patients. The goal of such a pilot project is to identify your challenges, including technical challenges, workflow challenges, payment challenges and anything else that might crop up. If this is your first video consultation project, you might not be aware of the specific issues that may go wrong in your business and the specific service you're looking to develop.

Every business and every service are different, so a pilot project can help you identify these issues. You can give yourself simpler goals than you would for a proper rollout of the service. For example, you might decide to do a couple of free calls for patients, so you don't have to worry about the payment side of things.

Advantages:

- You've created excitement – this gives you a fast way to move forward and do some experiments with patients, staff and clinicians and keep the momentum.
- It's a small-scale experiment that should help you learn more without having a big impact when (or if) things go wrong, so this reduces risk for your business.
- You're starting to set expectations with your clients – if it's successful, they will want it to continue.

Disadvantages:

- You're starting to set expectations with your clients and staff – if things go wrong, it might be waved off as a failed experiment and there might be less resistance to do the full transformation project.
- You might not actually get to test all the things you need to test in the limited setup.
- You already need to prepare a lot of things that you will also have to prepare for a full-service setup – it may not be worth your time doing it twice.

Set expectations

If you have no experience at all with video calls, running a small pilot is a good way to get some experience. If you do, make sure to let everyone know that you are doing a pilot and that you're doing it to learn about the needs for introducing a proper service. This way, people will not expect a perfect solution and are happy to contribute their feedback and ideas without getting upset. It's all about managing expectations.

What you need for a pilot:

- **Staff:** support for the pilot by your practice staff. You will have spoken with them for a couple of weeks by now, so they should be ready. We'll talk about this later in Section 4.
- **Clinicians:** at least one clinician to undertake the video consultations. Make sure the clinician's professional indemnity insurance covers for telehealth video sessions.
- **Patients:** at least one patient to hold a consultation with. Get the consent of every patient in writing that they are taking part in a video consultation trial and that they accept this approach for this particular session. If the patient is located outside Australia, you will want to check whether the clinician needs to be registered by the medical regulator of that jurisdiction to provide services there (see Medical Board of Australia advice on this: http://www.medicalboard.gov.au/Codes-Guidelines-Policies/FAQ/ Information-interjurisdictional-technology-consultations.aspx.
- **Hardware:** a computer, a video camera, microphone and speakers/headphones both for the clinician as well as the patient. This could also be a mobile phone or tablet, particularly at the patient end.

- **Software:** video calling software – you can do these pilot consultations using Skype, just be aware that it's not a professional solution with limited interaction functionality and security. We recommend using a professional health consultation software such as Coviu instead, particularly if your service focuses on more complicated interactions, such as an analysis of skin anomalies, or an eye exam. In such instances you will need to make sure your technology setup is much more sophisticated, and your pilot will likely focus more on testing the technical setup than some of the other dimensions. We'll talk about software requirements later in Section 5.
- **Network:** an Internet connection both at the clinician's and patient's ends and sufficient bandwidth to connect. More than 1Mbit per second up- and down-stream is recommended for good-quality modern video calling software. You can use https://www.speedtest.net/ to test bandwidth.
- **Booking:** an appointment between the patient and clinician. Before the first consultation, you'll want to do a test run with the patient to check their setup.
- **A decision on what to do about payments:** the easiest approach for a pilot is to not charge – but then somebody has to cover for it. If you decide to charge and you cannot use Medicare for (partial) reimbursement, maybe just charge the patient the gap that you would charge them if it was an in-person consultation. You might ask the patient to pay this at their next in-person visit to simplify the payment process for the pilot.

You'll notice that even a pilot needs a fair bit of preparation. To remove further challenges, you could do a first video test with family or friends instead of actual patients.

QUICK EXERCISE

Think of the different steps you will want to go through to get confidence you're on the right track: a video call with family or other clinicians, a pilot with patients, a full-service rollout. Write down some thoughts relevant to your case.

18

DIMENSIONS OF CHANGE: PEOPLE, PROCESSES, TECHNOLOGY AND A NEW SERVICE NAME

A service name

It's important that people can refer to your new service with a specific name and not just "that video service that practice x offers". Have a little fun with your new service and give it a title that you can use internally and with patients – it makes it more approachable. Think about who you're targeting and what disease and maybe have a play on words. This will also end up being your project title.

A project in Arkansas offering obstetric care to rural women called itself "ANGELS" which is an acronym for "Antenatal & Neonatal Guidelines, Education and Learning System". Another in New Hampshire for palliative care was called "ENABLE" for "Educate, Nurture, Advise Before Life Ends". One in South Dakota was called "eCARE" – a virtual healthcare hub that offered collegial support to rural providers for specialty care. In Oregon, a preventative dental care program that connected into schools was simply called "Virtual Dental Care" and a diabetes patient program in North Carolina that would offer access to an offsite diabetes care team was called "TeleTEAM".

You could include your practice's name in the moniker of the new service and make it a bit personal. You might be surprised about how a good name for a project or service makes it easier for people to participate.

Impact dimensions

When preparing to transform your business for a new digital service, these dimensions of your business will have to adapt:

- **People:** including staff, clinicians, patients.
- Processes: including workflow, support, digitising in-call documents.
- **Technology:** including software, hardware, networks, integrations.
- **Promotion:** including all patient material, marketing, listings.

- **Reimbursement:** including Medicare, payment gateways, other funding.

All of the changes have to happen in the context of legal and regulatory settings:

- Australian Privacy Principles: encrypted calls.
- All normal laws and principles still apply.

A project plan that is developed as the vehicle to introduce the new service has to take these dimensions of change into account and plan for their change. The changes need not be radical, but you cannot ignore any of these dimensions if you want to make a sustainable change. We're going to look at all of these dimensions in this section.

QUICK EXERCISE

What name can you give to your new service and the project you're preparing? Pick something that will get people involved.

19

UNDERSTANDING WHERE YOUR BUSINESS IS AT RIGHT NOW

Assessment

Before we can prepare a project plan that will introduce change, we have to assess where your business is at right now. There are some conditions that make it simpler to introduce video consultations than others. Assessing the level of sophistication of your business will give you an understanding of how much effort and money will go into introducing your new service.

Assess technology

Let's start with technology: how much has your practice embraced digital technology to date? Are you using a practice management software that manages patient appointment bookings and patient data records? Do you have current computers in your treatment rooms and for admin? Are they on the Internet? Do you have a public website through which patients may find you and book appointments? Do you communicate frequently with your patients via email, possibly even SMS?

Missing any of this is not a show-stopper, but it will make your project more extensive and more expensive, since you'll have to set up some basic digital infrastructure. You will at minimum need a computer connected to the Internet. We discourage practices from using phones or tablets unless absolutely necessary because it's harder to run a high-quality consultation from a smaller screen with less document-sharing capabilities. For a pilot or for exceptional situation – such as a doctor on the move between locations – smaller devices are of course acceptable.

Assess people

Next let's look at people: is your practice staff computer-savvy? Are they comfortable with digital technology and ready to try out something new? What about your clinicians? Is there an advocate amongst your clinicians who is happy to drive things forward, be part of your pilot experiment, decide on requirements and help write documentation and training material for the others? How about your patients? Are they families that embrace new technology or are they mostly part of an older generation that is still not comfortable with technology?

Again, none of this is problematic – you just have to be prepared to approach the situation with different solutions. For example, if you're dealing with elderly people who have never owned a computer, you may need to recommend a device to them (e.g. an iPad or an Android tablet) and may even need to offer them a tech support service to install the right app. Your technology partner may even offer you an ability to buy pre-installed ready-to-use tablets that you can rent out to your patient population for weeks at a time while they need therapy.

Assess processes

Next, we'll look at medical processes of your selected service: can that service easily be held online? What I mean by that is whether this type of consultation needs a lot of clinical tools to be delivered and whether the patient needs access to the clinical tools. If that's the case and none of your clinical tools are in digital format so can't be shared online, you may need to include a digitisation process at the beginning of your project. This typically happens in document-heavy specialisations such as speech pathology, where assessment tests and stimulus material needs to be shared with the patients.

What about the administrative processes in your practice? You'll probably want to start with having patients book video consultations just by phone as most of your bookings are done today. However, over the coming years, an increasing number of patients will start booking their appointments online via an app or via your website. Is this something you'd like to do from the start? It might help reduce any additional administrative overhead, but it will also increase the technology needed to start the project. Have a chat with your technology provider about these features and what they are able to offer.

We've found that most practices need to train up an administrative person to take on the role of "telehealth coordinator" for their practice. They deal with appointment bookings, make sure patients' technology works and they can video call into the practice, and help debug any high-level technical issues. For any technical issues that go beyond their capabilities, your technology partner should be able to provide in-depth technical support.

Over time as a practice and their patients become more proficient in video consultations, the role of "telehealth coordinator" may become superfluous. But it's often vital to set up recurring sustainable telehealth businesses.

Assess promotion

Next let's look at promotion: how much electronic communication do you already have with your patients? Do you collect their emails? Do you send regular newsletters? How about getting new patients? Are you on any listings? Are you doing online appointment bookings? Are you running ads anywhere? Have you maybe got a list of rural clinicians that want to connect their patients with your service? Or a list of patients that want your services?

If you are a complete newbie when it comes to digital communication and marketing, that's ok. Even if you already have some of this in place and can start connecting with patients straight away, there is – at minimum – some work to be done with explaining your new service. You will want to build a mailing list and promotion material as you go through your pilot project and not leave it all the way to the end for the launch.

Assess payments

Finally, you'll want to consider where your practice stands in relation to payments. Are your payments already managed digitally, e.g. through a HICAPS machine hooked up to your practice management and Xero? If not, you may be able to set up an online payment system just for your online consultations. In either case, you should ask your video consultation technology partner to hook up payments for online consultations in the best possible way for your practice needs. You will not want to have to send out paper invoices and chase your patients for payments if you can avoid it. A digital integrated system will also be able to also deal with Medicare reimbursements for your patients in the cases where reimbursement is supported.

Break down complexity

Thinking about your project from the basis of where your practice is right now allows you to get an understanding of the complexity of the project you are envisaging. Don't be deterred by any of this. Keep reading through the next chapters to create a rough project plan and a more accurate effort estimate before you worry about the involved effort. And remember: keep it as simple as possible so you can get some quick wins.

QUICK EXERCISE

Thinking about your project from the basis of where your practice is right now, what are some of the things that worry you? It's good to capture these as they are topics to discuss with your technology provider.

20

WHO IS RESPONSIBLE FOR THE PROJECT

Project leader

To run a successful transformation project, you need to know who is leading the project. This is the person that makes sure the project plan is executed. It could be an external person, but he or she needs the support of management to be able to get the time they need from the clinicians and admin staff to train them up and book them in for consultations.

Role of the business owner

This far we've made an implicit assumption that you as the reader of this book are the one preparing the project plan and leading the execution. We've further assumed that you are either the owner or manager of the healthcare business or that you have the full backing of the owner to undertake the project.

None of these assumptions have to be true. You might be a clinician in a healthcare business having an idea for a new video consultation service your business should introduce. Or you might be an admin person in the business who has heard from patients a frequent need for less travelling and would like to see the introduction of a new digital service.

Even if you are the owner or manager of the business, you might only decide that such a service needs to be introduced, but not actually do the project planning and execution yourself.

Project responsibility

Who is the best person to be responsible for owning the project execution?

The person responsible for the execution is always the business owner. They are the ones deciding what goes on in their business and have to accept that kind of responsibility. So, if that's not you, make sure you get their approval to move forward with it.

Project execution

Who is the best person to actually execute the project plan as the project leader?

This should be the person that is most passionate about it and quite possibly initiated the whole idea. This is the person who is best positioned to get everyone else excited and involved. If that person can't do it, they should at least be involved in the project execution and work with the one running it, be that an external consultant or an internal project manager.

Project pitching

If the business owner and practice management are not the originator of the idea, you will need to convince them of the project. This will require good preparation, including a draft project plan. Topics you will further have to cover with them are:

- **Service design:** which services – after hours, on demand, every Friday.
- **Patients to target:** local/remote ; target disease(s); target age group; target challenge.
- **Clinicians:** who is proposed to be involved; time effort.
- Staff: who is proposed to be involved; time effort.
- **Project budget:** what expenses are required, e.g. software, hardware, bandwidth.
- **Financial sustainability:** reimbursements, self-pay/gap, grant.
- **Proposed project plan:** steps and timeline.

Once they hear your full plan, they will be in a position to buy into it and agree to the project.

You'll notice we've already considered most of the information for the project pitch in the previous chapter that talked about the vision. Pitching your project is a way to get all that information together in a presentation and get buy-in.

21

PREPARING A PROJECT PLAN AND DELIVERY TIMELINES

Why do planning

A transformation project is like any other project: it needs a plan of what **steps** you are going to go through that will take you through to your goal, the **size** of the undertaking, what **time** you will give to achieve each of the steps, and what the **outcome** should be. You want to create a project plan because otherwise you're just stumbling along aimlessly, setting unrealistic expectations and confusing people around you.

Planning gives you a process through which to succeed and a way to judge whether you've been successful. A project plan doesn't have to be complex. If you are a sole trader, you will quite possibly be able to write it out now. The more people are involved, the more comprehensive you have to plan.

Go back to your project book. You've already designed the service you're going to start video consultations with in the last Section. Now you need to think about how you're going to convert it into reality.

Multiple projects

You might want to first plan a pilot and then a full rollout. We've already spoken about the pilot in Ch17; the steps for a full roll-out are very similar to the steps you go through in a pilot, except you have to deal with more participants and more complexity, so you will need structure, more documentation and more standardised processes. You can also have several such project rounds. There could be an internal trial first without patients before the pilot, then the small pilot, then a rollout project to a single practice, then a full rollout to all your practices if you're in a multi-location practice. It's up to your specific circumstances to define an approach that will give you the best chance of successive learning, cause the least disruption to your business, and thus offers the best chance of success. Small steps are always the best (see Chapter 47).

Example project plan

Here is an example project outline you can use to create your own project steps. Every phase – initial trial, pilot and full rollout – will need to go through a series of steps like these:

0. Project preparation:

- Do your research: goals of the project, revenue potential, number of participants for project.
- Prepare a draft project plan: steps and timelines.
- Make sure you have management support and any required funding.
- Be aware of regulatory and legal requirements e.g. around patient privacy.
- Check clinicians' professional indemnity insurances cover for video consultations.

1. Internal project kick-off:

- Identify project lead.
- Identify clinicians taking part in the project.
- Identify admin staff taking part in the project, including who will take support calls, telehealth coordinator, and technical support.
- Communicate project goals to everybody, e.g. through a one-page flyer about the project.
- Refine project plan in a kick-off meeting with participants, confirm steps and duration of steps, and distribute tasks.
- Discuss reimbursement approaches.
- Discuss promotion and marketing.
- Determine technology partner/solution provider.

2. Technology setup:

- Make sure participating clinicians and admin staff have a working computer on a sufficient Internet connection, a high-quality video camera, microphone, speakers and headset; minimise disruption by working with your IT provider.
- Determine which video-calling software to use via trials, then purchase and configure it.

- If necessary, determine how to take patient payments; you might need to set up a digital payment portal or maybe your solution provider has this functionality built-in.
- Determine how to take appointment bookings; you might need practice management software integrations for this or just start with phone bookings.
- If necessary, work with clinicians to digitise any material required within a consultation.

3. Training:

- Prepare training notes for clinicians and staff, e.g. through a one-page flyer with relevant instructions on how to use the technology.
- Set up training sessions for clinicians and staff; prefer times where they are not busy and will not be interrupted.
- Hold training sessions by running clinicians and staff through the whole process of how a patient books a video consultation, how the video consultation ends up in a clinician's calendar, how the patient and clinician enter a video call, and what can be done in the video call.
- Make sure every single clinician and staff gets hands-on experience with the setup, e.g. by having them do trial bookings and calls amongst each other – there are some skills to acquire to do a video call well.

4. Run sessions:

- Prepare service introduction notes for patients, e.g. through a one-page flyer with relevant instructions on how to book a video appointment and how to hold it, or through an explainer video.
- Prepare a questionnaire for both patients and clinicians to be answered at the end of sessions – this will give you feedback about what goes well and what went wrong.
- Launch service.
- Recruit patients for the video sessions, explain the required technical setup and get them to do a trial calls with admin staff for training.

- Get written consent from the patients for the video consultation sessions and get them to fill any forms required for Medicare reimbursement.
- Book video consultation sessions.
- Hold video consultation sessions and don't forget to require answering the questionnaire at the end of the session for feedback; some of these sessions should be accompanied by an observer to gain more insights.
- Run for a couple of weeks at minimum until you have enough feedback, possibly fixing fundamental issues along the way.

5. Review project outcomes:

- Review feedback provided by patients and clinicians.
- Collect required improvements.
- Is this now an established service in your practice? If so, you will need to think about how to continue attracting people to this service, e.g. through marketing, advertising, partnerships, listings.
- Decide whether to run another project to improve on the current setup.

Gantt chart

Once you're decided on your project phases and determined the steps in each phase as well as the number of participating clinicians, staff and patients along with the number of sessions you're targeting, you can start calculating time frames for each step. Now you are ready to create a Gantt chart that will help you calculate the duration of your project from these steps. It will look something like this:

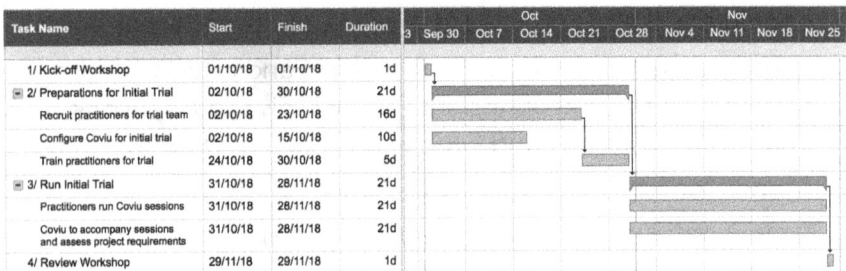

Task Name	Start	Finish	Duration
1/ Kick-off Workshop	01/10/18	01/10/18	1d
2/ Preparations for Initial Trial	02/10/18	30/10/18	21d
Recruit practitioners for trial team	02/10/18	23/10/18	16d
Configure Coviu for initial trial	02/10/18	15/10/18	10d
Train practitioners for trial	24/10/18	30/10/18	5d
3/ Run Initial Trial	31/10/18	28/11/18	21d
Practitioners run Coviu sessions	31/10/18	28/11/18	21d
Coviu to accompany sessions and assess project requirements	31/10/18	28/11/18	21d
4/ Review Workshop	29/11/18	29/11/18	1d

I recommend creating a raw Gantt chart for yourself, even if you are doing it on a piece of paper. It gives you a better understanding of the intermediate milestones you want to hit and the timeline your project will take. Since we don't want to interrupt an existing business, we need to be careful of how to add a new service and a good plan and Gantt chart reduce our risk substantially.

There is a lot of software available that lets you prepare such Gantt charts. There are templates for this in MS Excel, but I've found them to be too much work. There's also MS Project, which is particularly good for planning large projects. If you're looking for a free tool, I've successfully used SmartSheet (**https://www.smartsheet.com**). There are many others available – it's worth having a look around and finding something that you like.

Now, all you need to do is plug your project steps into the Gantt chart, determine a project start date and work from the first step through to the last entering their durations. You might even go into detail on the different tasks in the steps to get a better understanding of why a step takes a certain number of days. Plugging in dependencies gives you a way to build a plan that can easily adapt when a step or task takes longer than expected.

Manage expectations

I can guarantee, you will be surprised by how long it will actually take to run a project phase from beginning to end – and how long it will take to reach a sustainable service. That's ok – it's better to be realistic from the start and set the right expectations than to go at it uninformed and get disappointed when it doesn't succeed quickly. This manages your own expectations as well as those of others.

QUICK EXERCISE

Get your project book out and put together your project plan(s): sketch out different projects (trial, rollout) and the different steps in the project and list some tasks to undertake in the steps. Once you're happy with your sketch, create a Gantt chart. Write down any uncertainties about your plan below – it will be good to discuss these with your peers and obtain resolutions for your project plan.

22

WHAT DOES PROJECT SUCCESS LOOK LIKE AND HOW DO YOU MEASURE IT?

Why measure

Don't dismiss this chapter! Defining target metrics for your project is one of the most important things you will want to prepare before starting. Otherwise you work hard through the project and spend a lot of time but are unable to decide at the end whether what you've done was successful.

I've seen practices that decide to try out video consultations with initial commitment – often because they just had a patient who lives a long distance away in a rural area where they weren't able to get access to the practice's speciality. The practice gets set up with technology, holds a couple of video consultations with their new patient, but once this patient has had their therapy sessions, they stop with video consultations. Was this a failed experiment or a success? They don't really know, because they haven't collected the data. They might not even have asked the patient if it worked for them or not.

What to measure

Some of the things you could measure and put targets on are:

- How many patients took part in the trial?
- How many sessions were held online?
- How long does it take to a recruit a patient?
- Number of administrative complications encountered, e.g. with getting paid, getting meetings set up.
- Number of no-shows in comparison to number of no-shows in face-to-face sessions.
- Percentage of online sessions that went longer than planned.
- Percentage of patients that said they want to continue having this service.
- Percentage of clinicians that said they want to continue providing this service.

- Number of complaints about video consultations by staff.
- What percentage of planned sessions were cancelled because of technical issues? This is not just a test of the technology, but also a test of the technology-readiness of patients and their networks.
- What percentage of planned sessions needed technical support?
- Percentage of online sessions that resulted in the patient having to return for a face-to-face session.

Metrics for pilots

During a pilot or a small trial you may not have a very clear idea about what expectations to set on the impact-type measures. After all, that's what a trial is for. Most of your feedback in a pilot may be qualitative rather than quantitative, but you should still try to set yourself a quantitative target and try to reach it, particularly on how many patients are taking part and how many sessions are to be held. Once you have some experience and try a larger rollout, you can set yourself some of the impact targets.

How to measure

To capture this data, you will need to design a couple of questionnaires: one each for patients, clinicians and staff. Don't make the questionnaires too long – they should not take more than a couple of minutes to complete.

You can add questions with a five-level scale – a Likert scale: strongly agree, agree, neutral, disagree, strongly disagree. Such a scale has been proven to be easy to answer and good to quantize feelings. But also add a free text question so you can capture qualitative feedback. The questionnaire is best done online, which is particularly good for the patient and clinician who can be prompted at the end of the call. For online questionnaires, you can use a system such as SurveyMonkey or Typeform, or one provided by your healthcare technology provider.

What to measure

On every questionnaire you will need to capture:
- Patient reference: name, age.
- Clinician reference: name.
- Date and time of consultation.

You can also capture a code for the consultation, e.g. as a link into your practice management software where the clinician had captured patient data and consultation notes. But it might be best to also capture the details of the consultation, so you can associate results from patients, clinicians, and staff for later analysis.

Questions to ask patients that would be answered with a Likert scale:

· I was comfortable with the video consultation.
· I had no technical issues with setting up the video consultation.
· I had no administrative issues with getting a video consultation.
· I had good voice quality.
· I had good video quality.
· I was comfortable explaining my issues on camera.
· I felt the clinician understood me as well as they do in person.
· I was satisfied with my video consultation.
· Having a consultation online is very convenient for me.
· I would like to continue taking advantage of your online services.
· I feel compelled to encourage others to use this convenient form of healthcare delivery.

Also add: Would you have any other feedback about this consultation?

Questions to ask a clinician:

· I was comfortable with this video consultation.
· I had no administrative issues setting up this video consultation.
· This was an adequate means of delivering this service.
· The length of the consultation was adequate.
· The call quality was sufficient to provide appropriate advice.
· The patient has to re-take this consultation in-person.
· I had good voice quality.
· I had good video quality.
· I want to continue offering this online service.
· I feel compelled to encourage colleagues to pick up this form of healthcare delivery.

Also add: Do you have any other feedback about this consultation?

Questions to ask involved staff:

- The patient showed up to the consultation on time.
- Setting up this video consultation was easy.
- Setting up the patient for the video consultation was easy.
- There were no administrative complications.
- There were no technical issues with this consultation.
- I feel this service has really helped the patient.
- I feel compelled to encourage other practices to pick up this form of healthcare delivery.

Also add: Do you have any other feedback about this consultation?

You can also separate questionnaires for individual consultations from questionnaires for staff and clinicians at the end of the project. That way you can avoid repeating some questions.

How to evaluate

With Likert scaled answers, you will get a number between 1 and 5 as a result when evaluating your forms. You can also aggregate different questions that lead to a specific assessment, e.g. of technology or the acceptance of video consultations. You can therefore set your target for project success to a specific number, e.g. at least an average score of 4 for both clinicians and patients to want to continue offering video consultations.

QUICK EXERCISE

Make a list of the goals you'd like to achieve as a result of running your project. Think about the number of sessions and patients assessed, as well as results you can only get from questionnaires. Prepare some draft questionnaires while you're at it.

23

ADDRESSING REGULATORY AND INSURANCE ISSUES

Requirements

You will have to check out the regulatory, medico-legal and insurance aspects for your state and country before offering services online. This isn't really any different to offering services in person, but additional requirements may apply, particularly if your local healthcare system has different rules for states and nationally. This gets further complicated if you decide to offer services outside your country.

Situation in Australia

I'm going to take a brief look at Australia here, but please be aware that legislation changes constantly, and I am not a lawyer, so DO NOT take this as legal advice. I'm providing this information only to make you aware of some of the aspects at play in this space. This will be incomplete at best and at worst totally wrong by the time you read it. For up-to-date information please talk to your profession's peak body or regulation agency. You might want to start with the Medical Board of Australia's *Guidelines for technology-based patient consultations*.

As a baseline, your professional code of conduct and standards of patient care continue to apply for online consultations. So does your need to have a current professional registration – there is no specific telehealth registration. On top of that:

- **Duty of care:** clinicians are expected to make a professional decision about the appropriateness of video consultations based on each patient's circumstances – ultimately a patient's health is their responsibility.
- **Informed consent**: service providers are expected to acquire patient's informed consent and make sure that the online patient is correctly identified. In cases of emergency, consent is not required.
- **Confidentiality:** service providers are expected to protect their patient's privacy and protect their right to confidentiality – this is important since you need confirmation from your technology

provider that they can provide that kind of data protection. There are state and national privacy laws to abide by.

- **Accreditation:** clinicians are registered to provide services in the location of the patient. If a patient is located outside Australia, it may be necessary to be registered by the medical legislator in the jurisdiction of that country.

- **Reimbursement:** if Medicare reimbursement is considered, clinicians are also required to hold a provider and prescriber number from Medicare Australia.

- **Indemnity Insurance:** clinicians need to make sure that their Professional Indemnity Insurance covers video consultations/ telehealth services. Most of the policies of the major medical indemnity providers in Australia are broad enough that telehealth services are covered, but it's better to confirm.

There may further be specific codes of conduct, guidelines and policies for telehealth created by your profession's peak body – it will be good to check these out. For example, the ACRRM (Australian College of Rural & Remote Medicine) has a Telehealth Advisory Committee and it has defined a Standards Framework for dual care consultations, see: http://www.ehealth.acrrm.org.au/system/files/private/ATHAC%20 Telehealth%20Standards%20Framework_0.pdf

---

QUICK EXERCISE

The medico-legal side of video consultations can look daunting at first, but as you look into it, you will find that you are already covering most of the needs. Note down some of the things you want to check out and who to ask about them.

24

HOW TO MINIMISE DISRUPTION TO EXISTING BUSINESS PROCESSES

Starting a new business

If you are keen to build a completely different kind of practice – one that is just available online and provides no in-person services – you will not have to deal with the challenges of transforming your workplace. Instead, you probably decided to get together with some colleagues to form a new type of practice: an online-only practice. This can work well in some professions, amongst them psychology and psychiatry, dietetics and nutritionists. Anecdotal evidence shows that in these professions, patients are not actually all that keen to see their therapist in person – they often open up better about themselves when a computer screen mediates the communication.

Hybrid service

Most practices will, however, want to introduce video consultations as an additional service to in-person consultations. Transforming your practice to such a hybrid service offering can be disruptive if not managed well.

There are a couple of approaches you can take that will reduce your risk in disrupting your existing service and that make your new service successful from the start:

- **Buy-in:** if everyone in your business buys into doing the project, you'll get less people actively disrupting it and everyone will help when something goes awry.
- **Clarity of the service:** the simpler the service you are introducing, the more clarity you will get from everyone about what you are trying to achieve and to help you achieve it.
- **Small steps:** even if you want to introduce something complex, start with the smallest step you can imagine.
- **Well planned:** plan the steps and the goals well – a project plan as discussed in this chapter will remove as much risk as possible.
- **Clear directives (who does what):** the people that are involved

in the project will need to know exactly what to do and be well trained in what they are expected to contribute.

- **Telehealth coordinator:** in our many years of providing the Coviu service we have found that projects are more successful if they create a telehealth coordinator role with the responsibility to be the first point of contact for sorting out any technical and human issues around a video consultation. You'll need this role until patients and clinicians have become so comfortable with the technical that they don't need a human to help them any more when there are issues.

- **Integration:** if you can build the technology setup for video consultations into your existing technology setup and integrate with your existing ways of storing patient appointments and data, you can make the video consultations "business as usual". This is your ultimate goal.

QUICK EXERCISE

What are you afraid that the introduction of a video consultation service will do to your business? What risks are you taking? If you are creating a completely new business, what risks are you afraid of then? Take some notes and see what you can do to reduce these risks.

CHECKLIST: DO YOU HAVE A PROJECT PLAN READY FOR EXECUTION?

Re-consider some of the key points discussed in this section:

1. Have you decided on a pilot project?
2. Have you thought about key steps to execute in your project plan?
3. Have you made a Gantt chart to time your project plan?
4. Have you calculated how much the project execution may cost?
5. Have you decided who should be involved in the project execution?
6. Have you proposed what project success will look like for your pilot and the full rollout project?
7. Have you presented the plan to the business leaders and got approval to move forward?
8. Have you clarified medico-legal requirements?
9. Have you listed any risks that you're expecting for your business and how you may be able to address them?

4

We need to get everybody on board

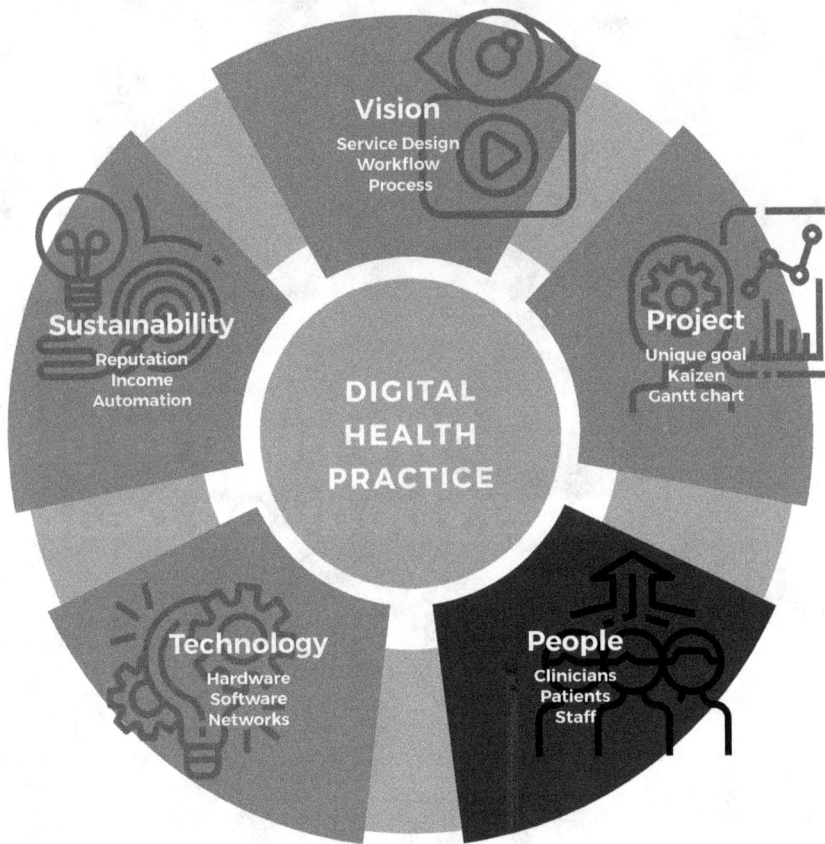

PEOPLE

In this section we're looking at the third component of the digital health transformation method: the human component.

25

WHO IS INVOLVED IN RUNNING YOUR BUSINESS NOW AND IN THE FUTURE?

Patient-centric healthcare

The modern view of healthcare is that the patient is at the centre of care and that healthcare is most successful when there is a partnership between clinicians, carers and family members around the patient that work together to achieve the best outcome. Your decision to integrate video consultations into your practice is likely driven by a future vision of your business that ultimately leads to such patient-centric care while being able to run an effective and efficient practice.

Your healthcare business at its core revolves around clinicians, patients and admin personnel. Let's for the moment consider the larger network around your patients and the potential that new technology offers to embrace this larger network. This goes beyond video consultations and is not something you will want to worry about when setting up your first video consultation, but as you become more proficient, you will find ways to support the patient better in their larger environment. In subsequent chapters of this section we will return focus to clinicians, patients and admin personnel, but let's think about the future for a minute.

Patient support network

Taking the vision of patient-centric care apart gives us an understanding of all the people that are actually involved in a patient's care. This goes beyond the players in your business, which are your clinicians, your staff and your patients. It extends on the patient side to family and friends and any potential carer or even other patients sharing the same illness. It extends to the pharmacist that provides the patient with advice and drugs. It extends on the clinician side to the patient's other clinicians – their GP, medical specialists, Allied Health providers, and the practices, clinics and hospitals they work in. Getting all of these to work together effectively and efficiently sounds like a healthcare dream come true.

It is technology that will indeed allow us to do so. There are now applications that provide effective and secure communication between clinicians that work at different healthcare businesses. There are self-help tools for patients and apps that provide continuous education for patients. We can have patients connecting with their clinicians as and when necessary. We can have digital records that are being shared between patients, their family, friends and carers. We can have electronically ordered drugs. And we can have multi-disciplinary case conferences by clinicians to jointly progress a patient. Technically, it's all possible, even if some of the technology is still very new. All of this has one goal: to move some of the responsibility about their health back to the patient, so they become more accountable.

Role of video consultations

Video consultations are one piece of the picture, but a pretty powerful one. Video consultations can enable patients to connect from their home and bring friends, family or their carer into the consultation. The same technology can enable patients to take part in group therapy, bringing motivation through shared fate and shared experiences. The same technology can also allow a patient to receive a specialist consult with their GP or pharmacist present for improved care. And it finally also allows multi-disciplinary case conferences of multiple specialists to discuss a more holistic picture of the patient.

Role of your practice

To make this happen in your practice, you need patients and their support network on board, you need clinicians and their peers on board, and you need the admin and IT support teams in your business to actively support processes and technology. A video call between a patient and one of your clinicians is merely the start to a more collaborative future in healthcare. It builds the foundation to much more – more capabilities of your team and more capabilities of the patient. In fact, it builds the foundation for a different way healthcare will be practiced in future – more partnerships around patient needs. You need to bring everyone in your practice along for the ride.

26

WHAT GETS CLINICIANS EXCITED?

Clinician opportunities

Some clinicians don't have all their time booked out. For those, getting more patients by seeing them online is typically not a problem – they have the time to train on the new system and ease into the new added responsibility. They probably also have the curiosity to try something new and work on their skills to become proficient in the new means of service delivery.

Busy clinicians

Most clinicians, however, have more than enough work on their hands. For them, adding a new way to deliver their services is a nuisance, no matter whether they are interested and curious about the technology or not.

The minute a busy clinician hears that they have to take part in a lengthy project and sit lengthy training sessions and have to use completely different systems than before, there will be push-back. That's natural because their focus should be on helping patients, not on learning new systems and processes. But you can make it easy for them.

Your goal is to make the new service a no-brainer for the clinician. The simplest possible change for the clinician – nothing to worry about – everything is done by the administrative people: appointments just turns up in the appointment bookings list and they click on a button instead of opening the door.

Minimise clinician disruption

Here are some tips to make this easy for busy clinicians:

- **Avoid wasting time:** don't make them take part in lengthy project planning meetings – maybe have a single representative clinician as part of the project planning group if you need it.
- **Up-front information:** book a brief one-on-one information and feedback session with them in their schedule at the start of the project, just to get their buy-in.

- **No technology disruption:** set up and test clinician's computer hardware, software and networks outside their working hours – make sure it works before their next appointment.
- **Minimise training time:** book a single short training time in their schedule just before actual patient sessions start, so they won't have forgotten by the time the first video consultation takes place. Make sure the technology is ready to go at that time.
- **Admin staff support:** organise all administrative details about video consultations for them, including patient bookings etc.
- **Telehealth coordinator:** provide them with a phone number for a specific support person to talk to for all video consultation issues.
- **Transition support:** get the support person to sit through the first (couple of) video consultations as on-the-job training. They should give the clinician helpful hints on how they can improve their consultation; they should also be observing any obstacles that turn up that make the clinician's job harder – e.g. if he/she wants to share any information flyers etc. These are issues to improve when moving from pilot to full rollout.

All of this leads to reducing, if not completely eliminating resistance by clinicians.

Turn clinicians into fans

Minimum disruption is a great achievement, but how do you turn clinicians into fans and get them excited about video consultations? You will need them as fans because they are the ones who will encourage patients to make video calls and they will talk to other clinicians and excite them.

Video consultations are a digital system – they should save them time and make them more efficient in the work they do. They should also make them enjoy practicing more because they can reach a much more diverse set of patients.

What you can do to get clinicians excited:

- Automate more administrative tasks:
  - Introduce a digital transcription of consultations, so they have to take less notes.

- Introduce recording of consultations, which gives clinicians more legal security around malpractice.
- Introduce online prescribing and referrals to reduce paperwork.
- Medical education:
  - Provide in-built mechanisms in the video consultation for clinicians to look up latest research.
  - Provide in-built artificial intelligence tools to help with assessments and diagnostics.
  - Organise participation in multi-disciplinary sessions with other clinicians.
- Patient feedback:
  - Share great patient feedback for motivation.
  - Try to get referrals of more challenging, more interesting cases.
- Clinician flexibility:
  - Allow clinicians to work from home to provide out-of-hours services.
  - Enable clinicians to take a patient's call while at a hospital or while travelling.
  - Offer wider flexibility of working hours.

Telehealth champion

One additional way to get clinicians on board is to identify a clinician telehealth champion. This is the clinician that is involved from the start in planning the video consultation project, makes sure that the clinician perspective is heard, and the clinician concerns addressed. They will know far more about the why behind the decisions made than other clinicians – why was a certain software chosen, why is a certain patient cohort being targeted, why is it taking so long to execute. They will be the communication mechanism to other clinicians who are keen to find out more. And they will be the encouraging voice that gets other clinicians involved and excited about the project.

Clinicians encourage your patients

As your video consultation functionality rolls out, your clinicians should start considering every patient that they see for video consultations. Not every consultation can and should be held online, but often clinicians don't even consider the burden they put on patients when requesting an in-person consultation.

When it becomes second nature to clinicians to first consider an online consultation for an appointment, that's when your project succeeds. The number of video consultation recommendations a clinician makes a week could indeed be counted as a measure of success. You could even make it a tally that challenges clinicians to get more patients on video consultations and creates some competitive spirit between clinicians for the uptake of video consultations. You might be surprised how well a simple public scoreboard can work. Just make sure this doesn't get out of hand – some consultations are better held in-person. Learning the right balance is part of the project.

It is necessary to determine what triggers each clinician's interest and happiness and then to try and give them more of that.

QUICK EXERCISE

Write down ideas for each of your clinicians – what might make them excited about offering video consultations?

27

INCLUDING YOUR PRACTICE (ADMIN) PERSONNEL IN DEFINING PROCESSES

Staff feel threatened

The people that feel most threatened by a change in your business are typically your administrative staff. They fear they are getting replaced by a machine. And to some extent they are right: you can run online consultations without having an actual brick-and-mortar practice and without any staff. When patients do their bookings and payments online and clinicians do consultations, referrals, prescriptions and initiation of charging online, what is there left for staff to do?

Need reliable staff

Let me tell you, unless you are a single-practitioner business and are closing down your brick-and-mortar practice, you will continue to need staff. You are better off keeping existing highly effective staff around through the transformation process and into the new service setup than having to hire and train new people about the way your practice works.

If you take the transformation slowly, as we recommend, most of your existing processes will need to continue to function – and they should function reliably. We want to focus our attention on the new process with small changes to the existing processes and not having to redo *all* business processes. A solid and reliable admin staff is your best basis to introduce innovations with.

Reassert staff

You need to address the threat that a digital transformation poses on your staff head-on. It's a communication challenge, because people are most threatened when they don't know what is going on, what is being planned, and whether their position is under review.

Turn it into an opportunity: involve your admin staff in your planning and process definition. Regard them as the experts they are about how your processes currently work, and work with them to define the new processes. They are in the best position to make the new processes least disruptive and make the transition as smooth as possible.

Involve staff in planning

This has to be done sensibly, of course. You can't just pull all your practice staff into a project planning meeting, and you can't give them tasks that will stop them from fulfilling their daily work. However, you can have a representative be part of your project planning team. They will take part in defining new processes and provide an opinion on what can work and what can't. They will communicate frequent updates to the rest of your staff. Just make sure they don't feel they are in a privileged position, otherwise they might make other staff feel worse about the changes.

If you don't have an obvious person that should be part of your planning team, you can even rotate and have different staff take part in the planning meetings. This way, you get a more rounded view from all staff, disrupt the work of the individual staff less, and make everyone feel included in the process.

If your practice has multiple locations, make sure you involve a staff member from each location in the planning meetings. Processes in other locations might differ slightly and require alternate changes.

Staff are experts

Let me stress this: don't treat staff as cheap labour to distribute unwanted work in your project meetings such as note-taking or meeting preparation. Instead, regard them as experts that you invite selectively and ask for specific input about the things you are planning. This way, they will feel empowered to contribute more valuable ideas. And when they have been part of defining the new processes, part of testing the equipment, part of discussing requirements with vendors, they will be in a good position to help update workflows, support communication with the rest of the team and prepare training material. They will be the engine of transformation.

QUICK EXERCISE

Write down some thoughts you have on how you can get your admin staff involved in the process, and who specifically?

28

CHANGING JOB DESCRIPTIONS AND INTRODUCING A TELEHEALTH COORDINATOR ROLE

Future job roles

The roles that you need to realise your vision of your future practice are likely to be different from the roles you need right now. This is the key reason why staff get anxious about changes.

Don't avoid addressing this challenge – it can make or break the success of your project. Instead, address it head-on even before you start launching the project. While the roles may change, the people do not have to be different people. However, they will need to do different work and that requires some flexibility for change.

Changing roles

You have a couple of jobs to do to manage this transition:

1. Define the new position descriptions.
2. Imagine who would do which work.
3. Work with your staff to coach them from their current position to their new one.

Start seeding the idea of the new service before you get too entrenched in its planning, and talk to your staff about it – this will give you an idea about who is open to change and who isn't. At this point, nobody should feel threatened, because you are still brainstorming.

As you become more concrete about the project, identify the new roles and come up with a draft of new position descriptions. If you're defining your projects well, the amount of change will be small and may just mean that a couple of people's jobs change marginally. E.g. a receptionist now doesn't just book in-person consultations, but also video consultations – or a clinician now occasionally holds video consultations.

Don't fall into the trap to think that your existing people will just manage. You really do need to write down a description of the new efforts. As you write it out, it may actually dawn on you that you are overloading a person with too much work and you may need to create new positions.

Telehealth coordinator role

We've seen that the most successful transformation projects create at least one new role in their organisation – that of a telehealth coordinator. They are responsible for solving all the challenges that could possibly go wrong with video consultations, including technical challenges, appointment bookings, patient data etc.

It sounds very similar to your traditional practice manager role, but has different challenges, so you could train your existing practice manager in this new role. If that creates too much work for them, you can always hire a different person to focus on this job. They will need to work closely with the practice manager(s) though because of their overlapping influence on schedules, patients, and the smooth running of workflows.

Eventually you will want to automate the workflows completely and have customers self-test their connection quality and ability to call in. So the job of a telehealth coordinator may become less necessary the more mature your video practice gets.

Transitioning staff

Once you have an idea of the new roles, imagine who would be appropriate for which role. Don't approach them before the project is solid but do have an idea who is key to success. You may be wrong about it, so maintain some flexibility. Ultimately, you can only decide by talking with your staff.

As soon as you have decided with management that the project will go ahead, announce it to everyone – you don't want the grapevine to create a threatening picture. Explain the big picture, the steps to get there and how everyone can have a role in it. Explain the advantages for the business, for patients, and the opportunities for staff. Get people excited.

Then organise meetings with every person in your staff to discuss their future role. If your organisation is large and has multiple hierarchical levels, you have to repeat team meetings on every level and follow it through by individual meetings all the way to the bottom of your organisation. The one thing you want to avoid is to spook your best people, because they are the ones that will be first to leave for another business if they feel threatened.

An analogy

In Cuyler/Holland's book *Implementing Telemedicine – completing projects on target on time on budget* they use a metaphor for organisational change that I quite like. It helps understand how important the human part of a business transformation is. They compare the change from an existing organisation to an envisioned new digital business to the change a theatre company makes when introducing a new play. As in organisational change, the people in a new theatre play will mostly stay the same, but their roles will change. It's a director's job to decide on the new roles and identify who fulfils them. It's a director's job to make sure that every person knows their new role well and has trained on it before the new play is launched.

Start thinking of your transformation project as a new play that you're putting on for your patients while giving your staff and clinicians new and interesting roles to perform. You will also have to be prepared to negotiate new contracts with some of your staff – if their roles change, their contracts and potentially their pay has to change as well with new responsibilities. You can compare this to hiring different actors for leading roles in a play – they will get different contracts and different pay depending on how important their role is.

QUICK EXERCISE

To get an idea of the roles you need in your digital business, write down the new types of work that need to be performed when your vision is realised. Then consider what roles your organisation currently has and who could do these new jobs effectively. Identify any gaps that may lead you to create new positions. Then come up with job descriptions for the changed and new roles.

29

TALKING TO YOUR IT PERSONNEL ABOUT VIDEO CONSULTATIONS

The role of IT support

We will look at the technology side of things in Section 5. Here, we want to look at the people side of technology: your IT support or IT personnel. This might be a contractor looking after your computers and software in your practice, it might be a medical IT support company, or you might be big enough to have part-time or full-time IT personnel.

No matter who it is, your IT personnel have to be involved in your transformation project. However, you should be careful when involving them to not let them run it. This is not a technology project. At the heart of it, introducing a video consultation service is a business transformation project and needs careful change management, as we have talked about.

IT support advice

Another word of warning: don't let the decision about what software to use be made by IT personnel. There is not a lot of understanding in the tech world about the needs of video consultation services and there is a risk that an IT provider will only consider solutions they are familiar with.

The minute your IT personnel finds out you're considering introducing video consultations, they will start suggesting all kinds of solutions. IT personnel are used to using video conferencing technology to collaborate with each other or meet with family members while traveling. They typically know a lot about consumer video conferencing tools and about corporate video conferencing technology simply because such corporate video conferencing technology has been around for a long time and has been used to save a lot on travel time in corporate businesses.

There is a temptation to satisfy video consultation needs in healthcare either through a consumer video conferencing tool (think: Skype or Facetime) or through a corporate video conferencing solution (think:

WebEx, Zoom, Polycom, or CISCO). However, none of these are a good match for a services-based business. You wouldn't use Microsoft Excel as practice management software either.

There are now specialised video consultation solutions in the market that are likely to be a much better fit for your needs, so when you get your IT personnel involved in the project, make sure to ask them to do a broad search and try out several solutions before suggesting a specific one for your practice. In Australia, for example, you'll find video consultation software such as Coviu or NeoRehab: in the USA there's e.g. Doxy.me, ChironHealth, MendFamily or eVisit.

Picking a technology partner

Often times there are customisations necessary to make the software integrate into your practice's workflows and other existing software systems such as practice management software. So it is good to pick a provider who can offer you such integration services and become a technology partner. They will need to work with your IT personnel to test and configure networks and computers during setup and ongoing, as well as maintain any integrations with other software you are using. Great customer support that can work with your IT personnel will be important.

You should get your IT personnel's support in creating a list of features your video consultation service requires. Then you can get their help in finding a technology partner that can satisfy these requirements, test the software, discuss customisations, discuss installations, discuss integration, provide custom development and support. Always remember though that they are there to solve your problem not to prescribe you a solution. The project lead, the practice manager, the clinician champions, the staff who understand workflows are the experts in defining a new service and need to be the ones defining the requirements.

Relationship with telehealth coordinator

Your IT personnel will typically help with the installation of the software and hardware and make sure that sufficient Internet connectivity is provided. They will work with the project team and the technology partner to set up the technical service environment and make sure the workflows work as expected. But in all the practices I've seen, that's where their work ends. Specifically, they don't get involved in user training, patient support, or first point of contact. They are not an integral part of the new service.

That is the role of the telehealth coordinator. They are at the core of running the new service and they will get back to IT personnel when there are technical issues around hardware and networks that they cannot resolve themselves. They will also get back to the technology provider if there are software or connectivity issues they cannot resolve themselves.

Let me repeat this because it is important: don't fall into the trap of making the introduction of video consultations a technology problem and giving it to IT personnel to execute. It is, at its core, a business transformation problem and needs careful change management.

QUICK EXERCISE

Think about when you want to get your IT personnel involved in your project and whether they should be involved during the project definition phase or only later on for help in selecting the solution. It will depend on your relationship with IT.

30

PREPARING TRAINING

Patient usability first

When selecting a software solution, one of the criteria will be how easy it is to install and use. The more user-friendly the software, the less effort you require in training. If it's too complicated for a patient to install and run without training, you will not be able to make this work as a business tool. Be sure to test the patient end thoroughly before deciding on a software. Entering a video consultation should nowadays be as simple as 'follow this Web link'.

You may still want to have an onboarding procedure for a new patient. It may consist of the telehealth coordinator sending an email to the patient to check their system setup and arranging a test call with them. Only when this has successfully worked will they be able to arrange a video call with a clinician. This can even be automated if your technology provider offers an automated test call facility.

Patient information

You will in addition want to prepare a one-page flyer about the service with instructions about the physical environment of holding a call in: it has to be quiet, well-lit with a light source not behind the patient, private without disruption by others, a camera setup that has the patient in the centre of the video, and any materials they need for the call pre-prepared next to them. Use simple words and keep it short.

You will further want to give your patients a brochure that explains the service, its goals, its advantages for them, how to book a video appointment, what documents are required before joining a video consultation (e.g. referrals), how payments work, what can be reimbursed, and addresses any other questions they may have, such as security, privacy and the handling of shared data.

Clinician training

Training of a clinician should equally be held to a minimum effort and again it's the software and integrations you set up that will determine how complicated it is for a clinician. If the video consultations are integrated into their appointment management system, it can be as simple as 'next appointment is online – click the link to enter the video consultation room'. If it's a stand-alone system, they may need to sign into the system first before being able to enter as a clinician.

Clinicians will want to understand the workflow – how the appointment is being set up, how the patient enters, how they enter. So prepare a simple diagram that explains how it all fits together and add that to a one-pager that contains similar information to the one-pager you send to patients.

Clinicians should only be trained when the system is up and works reliably to avoid wasting their time fussing around. Training should consist of holding a test call and focusing on camera skills – the use of the technology should take them only a couple of minutes to understand.

For clinicians, hold a test call with a real person at the other end and play through a fake consult. Understand what service the clinician will be providing and set the stage for them. This is a little bit like being on television, so the clinician needs to get used to it. Explain that they need to behave as they do in a face-to-face consultation: start with an introduction, confirm the patient they are expecting to see, make the patient comfortable with the consult, always look at them and not walk away off camera unexpectedly, provide good instructions and repeat them if necessary, speak slowly and clearly and always have a friendly look on your face. Giving just a little more energy to a video call than they would in-person helps make the patient focus and be involved.

Be prepared with digital documents that may need to be used in a video consult, electronic prescriptions if necessary, electronic referrals if necessary, and have the clinician explore all the features the video software provides, including scribbling on a whiteboard, sharing medical images, sharing medical forms etc. It helps if you record the clinician at the pretend-patient end and play that video back for them so they can learn from their own behaviour about how the patient sees them.

Staff training

Finally, your admin staff. To some extent, they need the most training as they need to be able to trouble-shoot. They need to understand what the patient experiences and walk a patient through any issues. They need to understand what a clinician experiences and be ready to remove obstacles for them. They may need to digitise paper documents that relate to a video consult. They may need to confirm video appointments with the patient and sort out any payment issues. They need to track that informed consent is given, unless the software provides for such tracking. They need to track that referrals are provided by the patient where necessary. Ultimately, they are the ones making sure the workflow is followed and is complete.

While I said "your admin staff", it may actually just be a small part of your admin staff that takes on these tasks – maybe just your telehealth coordinator(s). Also, the number of tasks they have to support depends on the functionality of your software solution. Some things may already be built in, such as the capture of consent, or patient payments.

It is useful for all admin staff to get one to two hours of group training about how video consultations work – then there is backup in case of sickness or leave, and it makes everyone understand how, for example, in-person and online appointments fit together. In any case, you will need to create a document of several pages that describes the process and how things are done.

Knowledge repository

You will also want a knowledge repository – maybe online – that captures the most frequently encountered issues – e.g. around hardware, software, firewalls, bandwidth, referrals – and how they may get resolved. A phone number of your technology provider's support line should also be provided in case high-urgency technical issues arise. This will be important for clinicians, telehealth coordinator, staff and even IT support.

QUICK EXERCISE

In your project book start sketching out the training brochures for patients, clinicians and staff. Train your staff first – they will help with the training of clinicians and patients.

31

HOW TO ON-BOARD PATIENTS

Lead patients

A lead patient is a patient who is excited about video consultations and keen to take part in the pilot. They will stay positive in the face of obstacles, continue to try and will contribute about issues. They will not be afraid of technology, will probably be quite technology savvy or at least be prepared to learn. They are the best kind of patient you can get to start a video consultation service.

To find such lead patients, you should talk to everyone who has patient contact in your business. Ask all staff and clinicians – they need to identify the right kind of patient that fits within the parameters of your project. For example, if you are targeting a new video diabetes service, you can only have diabetes patients in your pilot. Staff and clinicians will know which diabetes patients to approach to become lead patients.

If you cannot identify a sufficient number of lead patients, email all of the ones that fit the parameters with a request for volunteers. You might find there are some keen ones that your staff and clinicians hadn't identified yet simply because they had no idea about their circumstances. Maybe they lead a busy life – looking after relatives when they are not working, or working night shifts, or being on the road all the time. In such circumstances, going to a consultation is a challenge and just the idea of being able to take a consult from home is appealing.

On-boarding lead patients

Speak to these lead patients directly to invite them personally to the pilot. You can do this either via a phone call or when they are next in your practice. The invitation to take part in the pilot is best done by their clinician, because they are the person they trust. All the next preparations should be done by the telehealth coordinator or the project manager.

The telehealth coordinator should talk to the lead patients about their technical setup: what computing devices can they use, how to get to the software, and how they can test their bandwidth. It's best to have tech-savvy patients, but sometimes that's not possible, so you will need to do some "patient training". Maybe do a test call from their phone or tablet. If necessary, explain how they can share the Internet from their phones with their computer. This builds confidence and shows them video consultations will work for them.

The telehealth coordinator should also hand them a technical instructions flyer – not everything sticks when they have a chat with them. Or they could just offer to email them the flyer or a how-to video. It's important the patient can raise concerns, which is why a personal chat is necessary. They might be concerned about bandwidth use, about security, about getting an inferior service. The telehealth coordinator needs to address all these issues – and then make sure these issues are being tracked and included in future versions of flyers.

First consultation

As the telehealth coordinator finishes their on-boarding chat, they need to immediately follow up with creating the first video consultation appointment. If this doesn't get scheduled straight away, too much time will pass until their first online consultation and you will need to re-do the training.

Whether or not the first online consultation takes place successfully, the telehealth coordinator needs to follow up with the patient immediately afterwards. This is to confirm that everything worked, they can address any issues, answer any questions and make sure the patient felt comfortable with the result of the consultation. Make sure that either the patient or the telehealth coordinator fills in a feedback questionnaire after every appointment so as to capture data for the final assessment.

Expand patient group

To extend from lead patients to all appropriate patients in your practice, you will want to hang posters in your practice to announce the new service and put your brochure on display for the patients to ask your reception about and take home if they wish. You'll also want to email all target patients.

You can also post each target patient a letter with the brochure inside and an explicit invitation to join the project. A fridge magnet could be a nice touch to remind them this service is available and how to get their first appointment. You're probably best off having the appointments made by phone call because it allows patients to ask any other questions they may still have, and it gives your practice a chance to also create an appointment with the telehealth coordinator for on-boarding.

It may take multiple touch points before patients will try the service, so if you send out regular practice newsletters, it's good to repeat mention this new service you're offering.

QUICK EXERCISE

In your project book start sketching out how you can start getting patients for your project.

32

HOW TO ATTRACT NEW PATIENTS TO YOUR SERVICE

New patients

If you are targeting new patients to adopt this service, you will need to approach a broader audience.

Advocates

Your existing patients may become advocates and may refer other patients to you – encourage this behaviour by including a question in the feedback questionnaire about whether they would recommend the service to others and whether they have specific people in mind. If they provide names, you can offer to give them a brochure to hand out or ask for the referred email address or mailing address to send the brochure through.

Website

You will want to add information about the video service to your website. Make sure to include all the information from the brochure on your website and add a phone number for new patients to can contact you to ask more questions. You can also add an enquiry form that sends an email to you for you to reply. Be diligent with your follow-ups.

Advertising

You can put an ad into your local newspaper or into the local newspaper of regions you are targeting. You could even do a press release and call your local newspaper and explain that you are offering an innovative new service and whether they'd like to write an article about it – this way you can get a much longer information piece into your local newspaper for free. Alternatively, you could also get a guest article in a local newspaper explaining new technology and mentioning your service.

Content marketing

If you want to try getting patients online, you should post a couple of good articles on your website about your service and how it's making a difference to your patients. Explain a couple of the cases you were able to treat and the advantages that patients had from these video consultations. If you can get photos of the consultations and the patients, that's helpful. Testimonials by patients are also very helpful and build trust.

Consider creating a video about your new service and add it to your website as additional source of information. Videos often attract a lot of interest and help encourage people to call you for more information.

Social media

Once you have some content on your website, you can start reusing it to set up a Facebook page about your new service. You can even put a booking button straight onto the Facebook page if your software solution includes online appointment booking capability for video consultations. Invite your clinicians to follow your Facebook page and spread it to their patients. Post your case studies and other interesting information there, too. If you want to spend some money, you can boost these posts to get more people interested in your new service and book or call you.

Google business

To become even more proficient online, you should set up your business on Google (My Business at business.google.com) and explain the services you offer – it's free and helps people find you. This will help with your local business more than your online consultation service, but it does make people aware you have a hybrid offering.

Newsletter

Offer a regular newsletter that people can subscribe to on your website – it also helps attract new patients. The newsletter should be digital, though you can also have a paper copy for your existing patients that are less digitally fluent. The newsletter should include a description of what your practice does and why you are offering video consultations, any news of interest to patients about your practice such as opening times, possibly statistics about your new telehealth service, a 'Meet our Clinicians' section, interesting telehealth stories from other patients, quotes and testimonials from patients, photos and a list of frequently asked questions (FAQs) with answers about the telehealth service; here's a good example: https://telehealthvictoria. org.au/wp-content/uploads/2017/12/LRH-Telehealth-Newsletter-No.3_Dec-2017.pdf

Directories and listings

Register your online service with a listing service such as HealthDirect.

Partnerships

Try acquiring online patients in larger groups rather than one-by-one. This can be achieved through making a deal with a corporate who might subsidise their employee's health service because it saves them from having to take time off work. It can also be achieved through partnerships, e.g. partner with a GP clinic as an Allied Health services provider who has something special to offer, or partner with a rural clinic as a remote medical specialist service.

Measure success

Try to keep track of how successful each one of your efforts in gaining new patient is. If you find that most of your new patients come via your website, that's the best place to add more information and make improvements. If you find that your local newspaper ads do the best, continue doing those. Often it takes a mix of these approaches to get the best results, but measurement is always good. Ask every new patient how they found you.

QUICK EXERCISE

In your project book start sketching out some ideas for how you will attract new patients.

CHECKLIST: IS YOUR PROJECT PLAN SUFFICIENT TO ADDRESS PEOPLE ISSUES?

Re-consider some of the key points discussed in this section:

1. Have you considered all personas that will be involved with video consultations into the future, including family, friends and carer around the patient as well as team care?

2. Have you put together some ideas for how to get clinicians excited about video consultations and embrace it?

3. Have you got a plan for how to get your staff involved with the project?

4. Have you considered how staff work will change and who will look after the new telehealth processes?

5. Have you talked with your IT staff and gotten them involved in the project?

6. Have you prepared training for clinicians and for staff?

7. Have you prepared communication material for patients and a process to get them on-boarded to video consultations?

8. Are you planning to attract new patients to the video consultation service and if so, have you got any plans for marketing?

5

Getting technology fit for your workflows

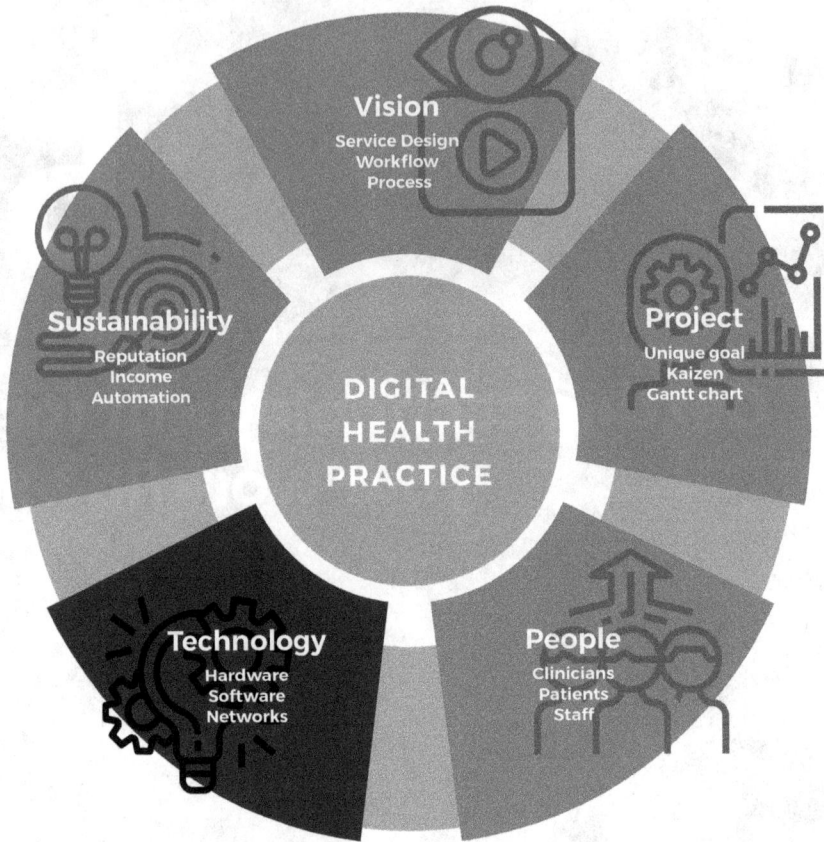

TECHNOLOGY

In this section we're looking at the fourth component of the digital health transformation method: getting the best technology setup.

33

ASSESSING YOUR CURRENT TECHNOLOGY STATUS AND WORKFLOW SUPPORT

Automation level

The technology you require to get started with video consultations depends on your existing level of automation in your practice.

If you start new or currently do everything by hand, paper and phone, including appointment bookings and the management of your patients' records, you will want to introduce a practice management software (PMS) first. This is a whole project by itself and requires purchase of computers and an Internet connection.

There are now many new cloud-based products available to choose from. I would recommend staying away from desktop installed software and go straight to a cloud-based solution, because it will save you a lot of effort in technical support and allow you access to your calendar and patient records from anywhere, not just from the computer where the software was installed. Pick a solution that is typically used in your industry and you can be sure that patient privacy and security requirements are being taken care of.

Seeing as you are looking for a solution that would work with video consultations, you can also make it a selection criterion that the PMS supports video consultations or integrates with a video consultation solution.

Technology dimensions

If you are already managing your patient records with an electronic medical records (EMR) system such as a practice management software, you should check a couple of things:

- **Computer:** to do video consultations, add a camera, a speaker, a headset, and maybe a document camera to your setup. The document camera helps with sharing paper documents into an online consultation.

- **Network:** to do video consultations, you need a decent Internet connection – we'll be talking more about the requirements in the next chapter.

- **Appointment booking system:** most video consultations are pre-booked, so you will want to consider an integration with your existing appointment-booking approaches. What software are you currently using? Can you integrate it with a video consultation solution?

- **Online appointment bookings:** if your patients are used to booking appointments with you online, you will want to check whether the system you use for online appointment bookings allows creating online video appointments.

- **Records management:** you want to continue holding your patient data in a single location, which is your EMR. Can you find a video consultation solution that integrates with your EMR and stores any data and information created during a video call back into your EMR? Can you store any video recordings from the online sessions back into your EMR?

Complexity of setup

During a pilot phase when you hold a small number of video consultations with patients, you will probably not have to worry about integrated workflows yet. For example, you can safely manage to take video call bookings by phone and add them to your booking system by hand with a note that this is an online call. Then take the online call with a system that provides you something like an online consultation room, preferably with a waiting room for your patient. However, when you decide to make the video consultations a standard service, you will want to consider a stronger workflow integration.

QUICK EXERCISE

Assess your current state of technology. Consider hardware, networking and software and list what practice management software your business is currently running on. This will be great preparation before talking to a video consultation solution provider.

34

NETWORK CONNECTIVITY, MOBILE AND DESKTOP DEVICES

Both ends matter

Let's specifically talk about network connectivity. Without network connectivity, you have no video consultations. There's your practice's connectivity and then there's the connectivity of your patients.

Practice connectivity

Your Internet connectivity at your practice needs to be sufficient for video consultations. This means that you should get a minimum of 350Kbps (Kilobits per second) upstream and downstream per video call that you want to hold in parallel. Some video calling software can provide video connectivity at lower bandwidths, but you'll get better results above this level. If you have multiple clinicians in your practice that want to hold video consultations in parallel, your bandwidth needs will multiply by the number of parallel calls.

On average, Australia's national Internet speeds are now at 9.6Mbps (Megabits per second) but this is downstream (for downloads). For video calls, you also want to be able to push your video stream up at a decent rate. The NBN (National Broadband Network) has plans with much larger upstream (or upload) bandwidth, starting at 4Mbps. If you cannot get NBN yet, there is a new service available in Australia called AnnexM which increases your upstream data rate beyond the limits of standard ADSL2+ and can achieve 1.4–3Mbps on your existing ADSL2+ connection. AnnexM is often offered at no extra cost by your provider, so find out if you can activate it to improve your video connections.

Wireless challenges

Something else to understand is that if you connect via a wireless network, your bandwidth depends on how far away you are from the base station. I've seen practices that organised video consultations to be held from a spare room at the back of the practice and were surprised to find that the connectivity in there was worse than at the reception where the initial connectivity testing took place.

If you're connecting via a wireless LAN from within a busy office, you might further find that the packet loss and the delays introduced by competing devices on the wireless make it impossible to get sustained bandwidth for video consultations. Make sure to test all locations where your clinicians and staff will connect from. And consider using an Ethernet cable connected to your Internet router to avoid a busy wireless network.

Home connectivity

If your clinicians are planning to connect from home or another location, they will also need to make sure that bandwidth is available from that location. This could be done via a 4G phone hotspot or their normal home Internet connection.

Corporate connectivity

In a corporate environment, such as from a hospital or a larger clinic, you might find that the network administrators have set up a very tight security for the network using a firewall. A firewall makes sure that computers from the outside cannot connect into any computer within your network without authorisation. This is a problem when you want to make video connections with patients. If that is the case for your project, you'll need to get your network administrator involved to set up rules on the firewall to allow such outside access.

You can test your network and a set of devices at **https://test.webrtc. org/** . It is based around the WebRTC standard that most modern video consultation solutions build upon. If everything goes red in the Connectivity section, you can pretty much assume there is a firewall in the way and you need to speak to your software provider about what changes need to be made to the network then hand that information on to your network administrator.

Patient connectivity

The connectivity of patients is another challenge altogether. Your telehealth coordinator will need to work with patients to make sure they can connect into your practice. No matter what device your patients are on – be that a desktop, laptop, tablet or mobile phone – they need to be able to connect to the Internet.

A patient may encounter lots of different networking conditions. They could be on a home Internet connection. If they only have an old dial-up line, they will need to consider alternatives, such as hotspotting their phone or using a tablet with a SIM card. An ADSL, cable or optical fibre connection on the other hand should typically be sufficient. For patients we suggest a minimum of 350Kbps (Kilobits per second) for a decent video connection.

Satellite challenges

Patients in rural areas of Australia are more typically connected via satellite. With satellite, you usually get sufficient bandwidth. However, the delay the signal gets because it has to go all the way up to the satellite and come back may mean that you have to wait quite a while to get a connection and to get replies from your patient. It makes for a less natural conversation.

Phone connectivity

Patients that are on the road or have no home connection can always use their phone to get a 3G or 4G connection. They may even share that connection as a hotspot, so a tablet or laptop can use the hotspot to connect. I once held a two-hour multi-disciplinary team meeting with several oncologists from a hospital over my 4G phone connection because the hospital administration had recently changed their firewall and had not provided firewall access to our software. The quality of the videos was brilliant, and we had no issues with the connection.

You can test a network's bandwidth and delay at **http://www. speedtest.net/**, both for patients as well as practices and other locations.

Bandwidth usage

A word about the bandwidth use of a typical video consultation for those of you that are concerned about cost. This is dependent upon the software you are using, the number of participants in the call (that's also called "endpoints"), and the bandwidth available to you. Most software will take up more bandwidth for videos if it can and reduce the video quality while retaining audio quality when less bandwidth is available.

Let's assume you have 1Mbps available both upstream and downstream. In Australia, your downstream bandwidth is typically much bigger than your upstream, but let's just assume that's how much we have available. Let's further assume there are two endpoints on the call (a clinician and a patient) and that the call goes for 30 minutes. Here's how you calculate your data usage:

Data Usage = 30 [min] x 60 [sec] x 1Mbps x 2 [users] / 8 [bytes] = 450MBytes.

Most ISPs (Internet Service Providers) provide you with a monthly quota, so you'll want to be aware of your data limits. For example, I have 10GB a month on my phone and I often hotspot it for video calls. My 4G connectivity is perfectly fine for a great video call. The two-hours multi-disciplinary team meeting that I hosted on my phone barely reached 1GB usage.

QUICK EXERCISE

Do you know the available bandwidth in your practice? Have you measured it at every computer where you want to conduct video consultations? Is it sufficient if all clinicians held a video call from their offices at the same time? What fall-back mechanisms do you have – any phone connectivity? Do your project patients have sufficient Internet connectivity? Do you have the right Internet plan?

35

HOW TO ASSESS YOUR SOFTWARE CHOICES

Types of solutions

When assessing what software to choose to support your video consultations, there are a lot of criteria to take into consideration. This includes comparing stand-alone video consultation systems with practice management software that comes with video consultation functionality built-in.

A fundamental piece of advice first: in today's world of cloud-based software solutions you should turn your back on any solution that requires you to install software on in-house servers or manage the running of the system yourself. Something like this may be useful for a large hospital with a large IT budget and a large IT department. For anyone else, cloud-based software should be the go-to solution. There are no ongoing software updates. Since you are using software hosted on a provider's servers, they will take care of ongoing updates and patches of bugs. There are no hardware purchases, hardware maintenance, hardware updates, security assessments, or lease of data-centre space – the service is run for you. To meet regulatory requirements, you will need to make sure your provider is Australia-based.

Other criteria you will want to use to assess your software are: functionality, ability to customise, usability, accessibility, cost, and support.

Features

Let's start by listing the functionalities that the software should provide. You will want to create a spreadsheet, list the features down the side and tick off whether a software provides for it or not. Don't value all features the same – in fact, you could just list those features that you know you will need and leave those out that you don't need.

Features fall into several types:

· Features within the video call: these are the features that support the patient-clinician interaction and may include things like video calls with 2-4 endpoints, group therapy calls (check the number of endpoints supported – an endpoint is a remote participant), shared viewing of images, shared viewing of documents, annotation of images and documents, shared whiteboard, screen and application sharing, sharing of document cameras and medical cameras, file sharing, note-taking, prescriptions, referral-writing, profession-specific tools as required by the clinician such as mental health questionnaire sharing, live view of heartrate monitoring data, or sharing of medical device data. Your service will not need all of these, but this list gives you an idea of what you may want to consider.

- Features upon entering and exiting the video call: these are features that are part of the administrative workflow and may include things like filling in of consent forms, Medicare card entry for reimbursement, private insurance details entry, credit card payment, any other kind of form-filling, entering a waiting room possibly with some entertainment, or being triaged by a nurse (or in future an artificial intelligence).

- Further administrative features: these are features that are required to get the patient to have a video consultation in the first place and may include things like online appointment bookings, patient detail acquisition, collection of a referral for the service, assessment of the suitability of video consultations for the patient's case, assessment of the suitability of the patient's device and Internet for the video consultation, filling in of consent forms, email reminders for the video consultation, or statistics about video consultations held.

- Integration features: integrations make sure the video consultation software is a seamless part of the rest of the digital tools being used in your practice. Integrations you may care about are integrations with your booking system, integrations with your patient records management system, integrations with your accounting system, integrations with your staff directory (Active Directory sync), single sign-on (SAML), or integrations with your marketing solution.

- Compliance features: it's a given that a video consultation software vendor needs to support patient privacy and security, is reliable and scalable. Depending on your country, there may be further regulations that video consultation software has to adhere to. In Australia it's the privacy principles. In the US it's HIPAA compliance.

Customisation

Next you should consider the customisation capabilities of the software. You may not think that you need to customise anything, but that's typically not true. There should at minimum be configuration possibilities to make the software work for your business. You may further consider whether the vendor is a good partner for you going forward with any custom changes that you may require.

Here are some customisation capabilities you might want to look for:

· Configure the pages the patient sees with your practice's branding.
· Configure the features that are available to a clinician in-call to customise to the profession and services required. For example, a speech pathologist will need different tools to a dietitian or a physiotherapist or an oncologist.
· Configure the administrative workflow that will take patients into a call, which also includes how appointment bookings are made and the setting up of integrations with other practice software.
· Availability of a custom branded mobile application.

You will want to consider how easy it is to make these customisations – do you need to work with the vendor or can you activate these yourself? The best systems have customisation functionality built-in.

Usability

Next you should consider the usability of the system. If a system is unreliable, not user-friendly, or too cumbersome, your clinicians will refuse to use it, your patients will try once and never again, your staff will turn patients away from it, and your IT staff will refuse to support it.

Here are some usability issues to pay attention to:

· How easy is it to invite more clinicians and staff to the software, and how easy is it to remove them again?
· How easy is it for patients to get into a call – do they have to sign up or is it simply a Web link they follow?

- How easy is it for clinicians to get into a call – can they just click on a link in their calendar? If not, can they just hang out in their online consultation room?
- Does it work in a Web browser or do they have to install software? Does it work in all major Web browsers?
- How long does it take to load the video call – anything that needs to install software and takes more than a couple of seconds to start will annoy particularly your clinicians, but also upset patients who are late for their appointment.
- Is the user interface clean and easy to understand?
- Is the process easy to follow for a patient?
- Is the workflow easy to follow for staff?
- Will the use of the interface require lengthy training sessions? Will it be cumbersome for clinicians to find the things that need to be done?
- Is it easy for IT support to administer the system?

It can be difficult to judge usability features, but don't underestimate their importance. If you need to find out how hard it is to get a video call going, do a test run with a non-technical person and see how they cope. Watch as they struggle through the steps.

Accessibility

Another factor to consider is accessibility. Any patient population you target will include people with accessibility needs. This could be older people, people with intellectual disability, people with physical disability, vision-impaired, hearing-impaired, colour-blind users, or a number of other users. Depending on your project definition, the likelihood that you need to support people with accessibility needs is higher or lower. Make sure that the software that you choose has accessibility features built in so your video consultation service will be inclusive of all patient populations.

Cost

The next factor we're going to talk about is cost. As a private citizen you are used to using Skype, Facetime or Google Hangouts for free. That's the one end of the scale. At the other end are corporate video conferencing solutions that include specific hardware, such as

Polycom or CISCO, where you can pay tens of thousands of dollars to get the video conferencing hardware installed. In between are Web based video conferencing system such as Zoom and WebEx. But none of these are actually tools that match the needs of a healthcare practice that uses waiting rooms, appointment bookings for a health service, payments and more. You will need to widen your search. Your cost expectations should be that specialised services such as Coviu or NeoRehab start somewhere around the same as Web-based video conferencing systems (which are around $20-$100/user/month) but can go much higher as the number of specialised features grows. Most platforms will charge per clinician per month, but other business models exist.

Support

The final important factor to consider is support. Since you are running a business based around the successful delivery of consultations, it is important that your video consultations all take place successfully and make you money. If something goes wrong, you will want support immediately and a resolution preferably within a few minutes. As you start out and do a pilot, maybe email and chat support is sufficient, but as you go into production, you will want telephone support. Expect to pay more for phone and video support – it is important for your telehealth coordinator to escalate any issues they encounter that relate to the system back to the vendor.

Consider your experience during the acquisition phase – has the vendor been responsive, are they approachable, have they been friendly, have they reacted quickly? It is highly likely that if your interactions during that phase were terrible, ongoing support will be a problem also.

You should also always ask for a free trial or proof-of-concept phase. Don't sign up for a 12-month commitment without having played with the software in anger for a few weeks during a pilot.

Extensibility

As you select your vendor, consider if you want to pick somebody who has a capability to make changes to their software system also. Sometimes you want a partner rather than just a solution, particularly if you are considering more challenging functionalities in the future that you've not yet seen in any other system. If you need a solution partner, get your IT people involved in the purchase decision and make sure they have a discussion about extensibility.

QUICK EXERCISE

Have you picked a couple of telehealth/telemedicine/video consultation solution providers? Go Google now if you don't know any. Then enter them in a spreadsheet and start making a list of features you'd like to see compared between the solutions. Also consider customisation capabilities, usability, accessibility, cost, customer support and extensibility as additional features to compare.

36

INTEGRATING VIDEO CONSULTATIONS WITH SCHEDULING AND MEDICAL RECORDS SOFTWARE

Digital conversation

Video consultations digitise the conversation between a clinician and a patient. Because it's now held on a computer, it can become part of other digital health systems.

Practice management software integrations

There are two fundamentally different ways for you to integrate video consultations into your digital health ecosystem: either you are using a practice management software (PMS) that provides integrations with video consultation software – or you are using a video consultation solution that provides integrations with a PMS or EMR (electronic medical records) system. In the first approach, your video consultation system needs to focus on making the conversation between a clinician and a patient the best it can, because the workflow features (scheduling, payments, reminders, consent forms, data storage, etc) are being taken care of by the PMS.

It is the second case we will explore further in this chapter. Even if your PMS integrates with a video consultation system, there may still be reasons to activate the integrations the video consultation system provides, e.g. when clinicians work at multiple locations or when the online booking flow of an existing system doesn't cater for location-independence.

Scheduling integration

The easiest integration is, of course, that with scheduling. This is a workflow integration. All modern practices use some kind of calendaring system to maintain the schedules of their clinicians. Since clinician time is valuable – no matter whether they are paid by the hour or by outcome – it is important for a clinician to manage their time wisely. With video consultations, this becomes even more complicated, because it introduces another "location" where clinicians are able to work.

Multi-calendar challenge

Let's say you are a clinician who is working on two locations A and B – A and B could be a hospital and a private practice or two private practices at different ends of town. Typically, you would divide your week between the locations and have staff at the two locations book patient consultations only on the days you are at that location. This makes it easy to keep the two calendars separate for the two locations.

Enter video consultations: suddenly it doesn't matter any longer what physical location you are in. You could be filling gaps in your calendar at any location. You could be taking emergency appointments for patients that turn up at practice A on days where you are practicing at practice B. If such a gap-filling use of video consultations is your aim, you will want to integrate all your calendars into one and allow your video consultation booking system to get access to your availability. It will then allow patients and the staff at locations A and B to make an online appointment booking by picking a time slot when you're free.

The integrations necessary for such a scenario are as follows: assuming you are holding two calendars, the video consultation application will then need to be able to extract availability from both calendars. It will then display availability to the patient, have the patient select a date and time, book the patient into the picked time slot with a specific service picked from a list of online available services, and communicate this booking back into the calendar(s). Technically speaking, this is typically done via an API (application programming interface) that both calendaring systems need exposure to, and an integration developed by the video consultation software company.

Check if your video consultation solution integrates with such booking APIs if you want to provide online appointment bookings and run a hybrid online/in-person clinic. You may be able to pay for the development of such an integration.

Payments

The next integration you may be interested in is with payment gateways. As you integrate online bookings, you may also want to integrate online payments for sessions via credit card. For this, your solution needs to integrate with a payment gateway such as Stripe, Braintree, PayPal or Square. And possibly with an accounting system like Xero or MYOB.

Reimbursements

If you want the video consultation system to help patient do reimbursements, you will want to check if your solution provides Medicare and/or HICAPS integrations.

Marketing

There are other integrations you may be keen to have, including anything to do with marketing, analytics and tracking the results of marketing, e.g. through Google Analytics or the Facebook Pixel. When you get to that level, you will know what you need from your practice management software.

Medical records

The final type of integration we will discuss is that with medical records. This is an in-call integration more than a workflow integration with patient information flowing from the EMR into a telehealth session and back into the EMR. The purpose here is threefold:

- To be able to pull up medical imaging, pathology and other medical records to share with the patient during a call.
- To be able to acquire any digital medical information that the patient shares in the video consultation into the EMR.
- To retain all medical documentation that is created about a patient in the EMR.

A medical records integration with a video consultation can be quite simple: medical imaging, pathology, forms and other records could be shared with the patient via a screenshare or document share, and all documentation the clinician does during the consultation is input directly into their existing EMR/PMS. Any documents that the patient shares need to be downloaded to the clinician, who can then add it into their EMR.

This is the minimum that is required to keep a unique patient record. It's important for continuity of care not to have records stored in multiple places for one patient, so this is an important process in which to train clinicians.

To make it simpler for clinicians, a tighter integration and automatic record update in the EMR is possible. This will require all documents and images that a patient shares to be added to their EMR record by the video consultation application. Typically, such an integration is done via a medical records file format like FHIR (Fast Healthcare Interoperability Resources). Similarly, documents that the clinician shared with the patient and that were annotated may need to be added back into the EMR.

A final step in EMR – video consultation integration would be to give the video consultation application direct access to the patient's medical records, so the clinician can more easily pull up and share the patient's latest imaging or pathology results for discussion. This streamlines the interaction and makes the clinician focus on the video consultation rather than having to jump back and forth between the video consultation and the EMR. It also leads to a more focused conversation between clinician and patient, providing the patient with a better experience.

Other integrations

There are many other integrations that are possible, such as with mobile apps that capture patient data, workflow systems, accounting systems, medical analytics systems, etc. You'll have to consider what systems you're currently using that you'd like to see supported in video consultations.

QUICK EXERCISE

For a pilot, integrations may not be at the top of your priority list. But when you choose a video consultation solution and try to integrate it with your EMR and PMS, it's advantageous to find out if the vendor is already offering such an integration or whether it would be possible to develop such an integration for your project. Take a few notes about what systems you would like to see integrated into a seamless workflow.

37

WHAT MEDICAL DEVICES AND TOOLS DO YOU USE FACE-TO-FACE?

Need for face-to-face

Only in about 20% of clinician visits does a clinician need to lay hands on a patient. Most of the remaining cases actually don't require the clinicians' hands, but either a medical device, or just somebody's hands.

There are situations where the clinician needs to examine a patient physically, e.g. to get their temperature, blood pressure, eye background or analyse cramped muscles. Such services can only be supported via video consultations if a local person can be the hands of the remote clinician and the local person has access to the kinds of medical devices the situation calls for.

Medical devices

But don't believe, just because you need a medical device to examine, diagnose or help a patient, you cannot provide this as a service to patients. The world is changing, and we are seeing a consumer revolution in the medical device sector. Many of the diagnostics and monitoring devices that used to be restricted to being owned by clinicians or hospitals are now available as mobile and wireless devices for the home.

Consumer medical devices

Think about wearable Bluetooth baby thermometers, digital wireless stethoscopes, wireless scales, wireless blood pressure cuffs or even simple pathology strips. There are many start-ups working on new medical devices and device packs for the home. Consider how families now own a thermometer. A couple of years from now, they will own a little kit of different wireless medical devices and mobile phone attachments that will be used when children are sick and need an urgent GP visit – why pull them out of bed when they can get the GP to join via a video call. Teaching consumers how to use the devices correctly is part of what the start-ups are doing, so suddenly, there are many hands that can be the remote hands of a clinician.

Clinicians need to be prepared to make that transition with their patients. If clinicians start gaining experience with video consultations for simple consultations now, they will be prepared for the future. GPs could, for example, start by simply providing referrals to a specialist or a prescription in a video consultation.

Medical diagnostics

Where more involved medical diagnostics devices are needed for a consultation, such as an otoscope camera, and ophthalmoscope, a spirometer, an electrocardiograph, a wireless hand-held ultrasound, video consultations that plug into such devices and remotely share the data with a specialist are still useful, because many of these devices can be handled by a nurse.

More involved monitoring devices are coming out also, such as uninterrupted cardiac monitoring (iRhythm), glucose monitors, blood pressure monitors, pulse oximeters, multi-parameter monitors and sleep apnoea monitors. This can now be installed in patient homes and call back to a clinician in case of irregularities or emergencies. If this is part of the service you want to provide, you will need to make sure that your video consultation provider also works with a monitoring device company.

Medical tools

Other things you need to consider when choosing your video consultation solution revolve more around the types of medical tools clinicians use during consultations, which are diagnostic questionnaires, charts, standardised tests, information brochures, and other stimulus material. You will need to be able to add these to your video consultation and the technology has to be able to enable this.

QUICK EXERCISE

Thinking about all the tools you use during a consultation in-person, consider what you need to replicate in digital form to be able to provide the best quality online consultation. Sometimes a local nurse or trained helper can give extra capability.

38

DOES YOUR PHYSICAL SPACE SETUP NEED ANY CHANGES?

Physical space

When you are setting up a video consultation environment, you should also consider the physical space from which you're holding the consultation. After all, this is a "video production" you are creating. Don't worry, it doesn't have to be professional, but if you follow a couple of ground rules, the experience that your clinicians and patients have will be so much better.

Incidentally, you will also want to notify your patients of these tips before they get on a call.

Light

Make sure the room clinicians are taking the call in is bright enough. You can check the quality in your video consultation software when setting it up and looking at your local video. If you have a bright window behind the clinician, you might need to get the blinds down or turn on the lights to shed more light on your face. A spotlight on their face can also help. If you are able to move the computer, it's best to position it away from the bright window or they'll just turn into a black shadow.

Noise

It's not easy to take calls in rooms with a lot of background noise. In such a situation, at minimum provide headsets and use the microphone of that headset also. That at least exposes the voice better to patients and decreases the volume of the background noise. If you are in an office, close the door and make sure staff knows that a video consultation is going on and to avoid disturbing it. Maybe even hang a sign in front of the door. Turn off any radio or TV that is running.

Distraction

Anything that moves behind the clinicians in a video call is going to be distracting for patients. Any moving toys, screens, or TVs need to be moved out of the picture. If you can't remove the things behind you, consider buying a portable screen. There are some very affordable blue or green screens available now that just stick to a chair and blend out everything that goes on behind the clinician. They provide for a nice uniform background without distraction. Some video consultation software even provides you with an ability to replace the screen with a randomly chosen background for the patient.

Setup

Make sure that all documents and data the clinicians need for the consultation is near their screen. The last thing you want is a clinician running out of the picture to pick up something. Similarly, all data needs to be available on the computer from which they are running their consultation, so they are able to access and share it during the call if necessary. You could even set up a second screen for the clinician, so they can put the video consultation on one screen and the practice management software/EMR on the other screen. This leads to an enhanced experience for the clinician who doesn't have to switch between windows.

QUICK EXERCISE

Do an assessment of all the environments from where a clinician will be holding video consultations and note down all the things you need to fix in preparation for video consultations.

39

WORKING THROUGH PLANNED WORKFLOWS USING CHOSEN HARDWARE AND SOFTWARE

Connecting the dots

By now you will have assessed all your technology needs and come up with a list of things needed for your video consultations. It's time to put the pieces together.

Design the workflow

Before you purchase the software that will turn your imagination into reality, make a drawing that shows the full workflow. Draw the workflow for the patient, for the clinician, the administrator and, if necessary, the IT person. These drawings will be good to put in front of your project team and confirm that this is a desirable workflow and that it will be workable. If there are any gaps in the workflow, you will need to get back to your technology partner to get them to quote you for the extra functionality required.

When you have it on paper, it's easier to check back later to confirm that your planning was accurate, which is a good learning experience for the next projects you're planning. You'll also discover what the typical things are that you neglected so as not to neglect them next time.

Testing the technology

If you are dealing with multiple software and hardware providers, you might be able to get a trial version of the software (or a free trial period) and sample devices from your hardware provider so you can try to put these workflows together to test if they will actually work. You can also compare the quality of the different devices and software products. This should help you make a decision about what to buy.

Testing the workflow

Finally, once you are satisfied you've found the best solution, you need to get it all set up and test again. This will involve more than just software, hardware, networks, and medical devices – it will also involve any forms, digitised charts and digitised brochures that clinicians use in their consultations. Make sure you test everything thoroughly. Don't just rely on your IT person saying that it works – actually get a trial run with a pretend patient and a real clinicians to confirm the setup is up to the task.

QUICK EXERCISE

Go back to your earlier notes about what a workflow will look like and make sure you set up your technology to cover all involved steps for patients, clinicians, admin and IT.

40

ADDING TECHNOLOGY REQUIREMENTS AND ASSESSMENTS TO YOUR PROJECT PLAN

Planning technology setup time

Now that you know what you have to do to set up technology, add the discussed tasks to your project plan and make sure to associate sufficient time to complete the technology setup.

Include the following tasks:

- Assess your technology readiness level.
- Assess your available technology and any gaps: hardware, software, networks.
- Assess your physical spaces.
- Define the assessment criteria for the software.
- Define what medical devices and tools you will need.
- Assess available software solutions and their providers to determine a technology partner: functionality, customisation, usability, accessibility, cost, support.
- Assess integration needs between systems.
- Define details on the workflow needs.
- Test and pick software and hardware.
- Define any extra software development needs.

Consider the order in which you want to do this work, how long each will take and their dependencies. You should be able to add this to your existing Gantt chart.

QUICK EXERCISE

It's time to add detailed steps about your technology audit, requirements, assessment and choice to the timeline of your project plan. Write it in your project book and take any notes.

CHECKLIST: IS YOUR PROJECT PLAN SUFFICIENT TO ADDRESS TECHNOLOGY ISSUES?

Re-consider some of the key steps discussed in this section:

1. What is the current situation of your technical setup? Do you use an EMR or PMS system? Are you on the Internet with sufficient bandwidth? Do you have video conferencing hardware? Are medical devices required in your video consultation scenario?

2. What are the requirements on the video consultation software that you need to acquire?

3. Do you need customisation of video consultation software and do the vendors that you look at allow for it?

4. Have you planned for the assessment of software and hardware in the market?

5. Have you planned enough time into your project plan to set up reliable technology to support your workflow?

6

Making video consultations sustainable

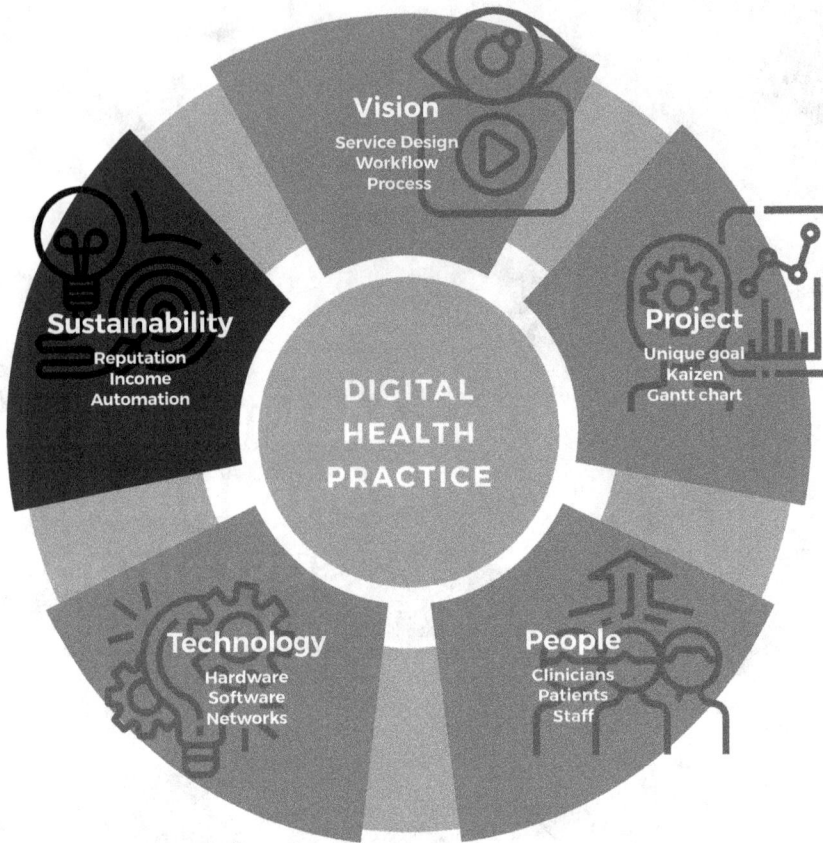

SUSTAINABILITY

In this section we're looking at the fifth component of the digital health transformation method: getting your service sustainable.

41

EXECUTE WITH CONVICTION: CONFIDENCE, PERSISTENCE, FLEXIBILITY

Optimism

Let's be realistic: not everything is going to go well all the time. There are going to be times when everything seems broken and nothing is working the way you expected. That's just part of digital transformation and you learn how to deal with problems and develop backups (such as a 4G connection as backup for the Internet being down). In fact, failure is part of any changes you make in life. If everything always worked as expected, that would be boring. However, that's not a reason to give up – keep pressing on.

The funny thing about the human psyche is that if you are convinced the problems can be overcome, everyone else around you will be convinced also and actively help fix it. Don't ever doubt that you may be on the right track – digital healthcare is coming, and you need to be prepared for it. Push through any issues and you will emerge with the kind of learnings that others are jealous of.

Flexibility

At the same time, don't be precious about your original idea on the kind of service you could offer. It may turn out you picked a really difficult service to start off with and you need to simplify your idea. So, be flexible with your execution.

Continuously learn about what works and where you get resistance. If your staff resist a change, analyse why, talk with them, make alternative suggestions until you find a way that people can agree. Be confident, persistent, and yet flexible.

Validation

Also learn from the pilot project(s) that you're doing – continuously test your assumptions. Talk with patients and get their ideas for what they would like to see.

A bit of a warning though: there will be lots of advice and lots of people telling you how you're doing it all wrong or how something will never work. Ignore the nay-sayers – unless they have real data and good arguments, they are usually wrong. You understand your business best. Take advice, but don't let it overwhelm you. Learn more from your patients and clinicians that are doing video consultations than from third parties that are just speculating.

QUICK EXERCISE

Who are the people that you want to listen to? Where do you expect criticism to come from? Who should you ignore? Write it down and when you feel stressed about the project and some negative input from somebody, get back to these lines and note whether you expected them to be a resistant.

42

BUILDING YOUR BUSINESS REPUTATION BEYOND THE BORDERS OF YOUR PRACTICE

Opportunity

There is a huge opportunity for you in video consultations: you can build your practice a reputation far beyond the immediate environment of your physical practice. This will give you a growth potential you don't have with a purely local practice.

Specialisation

For this to happen, it's actually best to focus on a very specific service for which you are simply the best. This is because you need to get word out and it's easier to be heard if you have a great story to tell and something very specific to offer. You have to be remarkable – as in: people will want to remark about you.

Spread the word

Once you have identified that specific service, you need to publish about it. After all, you want to attract patients to it. There are lots of things you can do, but some of the core things are around setting up an online website, writing articles about it, getting patient testimonials and case studies, publishing infographics and videos, writing blog posts on related sites, setting up a Facebook group, and getting your existing patients to help you get the word out. You might even want to approach the newspaper to write about your service, make press releases, put ads into local newspapers in areas you are targeting, get some radio ads, Google ads and even radio ads. Just be persistent. Even with a low level of publishing about your service, people will start to discover you in their Google searches and eventually word will come around.

Professional reputation

In parallel, you probably also want to let your peers know about your special service, because that builds your reputation, which in turn brings you more patients. Some things to do would be speaking at conferences and seminars about what you're doing, making scientific publications if you have some specific insights, write journal articles, talk to your industry association about featuring your work in their newsletter, write LinkedIn posts and create a podcast.

Differentiation

If your video consultation service is successful, your peers will want to learn about it. Don't hide your success – work it! Talk about how you did it publicly, because that will get you patients as well as attract clinicians with an interest in the space. You want to make the service sustainable, so use it to differentiate your practice.

QUICK EXERCISE

Let's brainstorm a little. What are some of the things that you'd like to do once your video consultation service has seen some success? How do you want to let patients know, so you can further grow the number of online consultations? Do you want to extend your practice's professional reputation as well?

43

THE BIG DAY – YOUR DIGITAL SERVICE LAUNCH

Internal launch

Launch day should be a big thing for you, but it may go completely unnoticed by most outsiders. It's the day that everything is ready, and you can start holding your first video consultations with patients. You'll probably have a video consultation booked for that day because that makes it real. When that takes place successfully, you can celebrate. Perhaps make a special cake and celebrate the day with your staff.

Service launch

We're making this a big thing not because of the video consultation – holding a single video consultation isn't that hard, after all it could just be a video call with a patient. However, this is a service launch and it should start you on a journey of sustainability.

As a service launch, you will have goals, plans, processes, and systems in place and all of these have been finalised at this date. That's what you are celebrating.

You'll want to tell the world about it – don't! Not on this day. You need to wait until you have a few successful consultations and a bit of experience. You need stories that you can tell. Do a retrospective at the end of the first week after the service launch to assess what worked, what didn't and what could be improved. Repeat that a week later until you're confident about announcing it to the world.

Public launch

Pick a day for your public launch that is a couple of weeks or months after you've officially started holding video consultations with patients. By this day, you should have most of the technology kinks sorted, you should have created the necessary brochures and marketing material, you should have a couple of success stories to tell, and you should have all your clinicians and staff on board and actively supporting the launch. You might make this a big day for the business – including a press announcement, a little party, launch of some advertising in the local newspaper, etc. This is when all your patients and potential new patients will hear about it.

QUICK EXERCISE

Don't underestimate what you have achieved by your internal launch day. Make a list of the things you will be proud of by that day. Also make a list of the things you want to have seen in place before your start telling others about it.

44

MAINTAINING ENTHUSIASM: COLLECTING AND SHARING SUCCESS STORIES

Amazing moments

A video consultation project might be a lengthy project going over multiple months. Sometimes things may not go as well as you'd like, but other times you'll get euphoric because something amazing just happened.

I had a customer once – a speech pathologist providing video consultations into remote Australian schools. She told me her story about a child that was slightly autistic in Year 2 of a rural school. The child had never spoken a word to a teacher or the other children. After having had a couple of video consultations with the speech pathologist from Sydney, something amazing happened: the child walked up to a school friend on the playground and repeated their name. Their teacher, students, family, and in fact the speech pathologist were completely surprised by this and deeply shaken by the fundamental change it had brought to this child's life.

Collect stories

It's stories like these that you want to cherish. Don't turn them into fairy tales – turn them into case studies that you write up and publish, share with other patients and consider submitting an article to a scientific journal or conference. Your learnings are valuable – take them seriously!

It's stories like these that will also maintain your enthusiasm in the project and your commitment to the long-term goal of a digital health practice.

Types of stories

Your stories might not evolve around a patient, but maybe around a clinician or a team member or an IT person. I once worked with a clinician who totally rejected the need for video consultations. They were technically competent, but just didn't believe that it was the right medium for healthcare consultations. After involving them more deeply in the planning of the project and giving them some responsibilities, they turned into the strongest advocate in the team. This is not a story you want to share publicly, but it is a story that can help you through challenging times in the project.

Progress

These stories will also be good arguments to lead from a first small project to a second larger project. Aside from reaching quantitative goals, stories are a second powerful reason to continue along a successful journey.

QUICK EXERCISE

Do you already have some anecdotal stories that might motivate you? How will you start collecting your success stories?

45

MINIMISING DISRUPTION: SUPPORT AND OPERATIONS

Smooth operations

A sustainable business is one that operates smoothly. To have a business with smooth video consultations requires minimising disruptions.

One of the most detrimental sources of disruptions of video consultations are when the video connection does not get created. This hits directly on the morale of clinicians, patients, and staff and has to be addressed immediately.

Tiered support

A sustainable video consultation service therefore includes an outstanding support service. This support needs to have multiple levels, getting increasingly more technical.

At first is the telehealth coordinator. They will help patients and clinicians with their hardware, software, device and network issues and rule out the obvious user mistakes.

The second level of support needs to be a technical person who can check more deeply. If they identify the source to be a software issue, they need to get the software provider on the phone. If they identify the source to be a network issue, they need to get the network provider on the phone. Hardware issues cannot usually be sorted out so quickly and may require replacing certain devices and machines.

With excellent support through the telehealth coordinator, most problems will be addressed quickly and a call that may not have started in the first couple of minutes will still be able to take place.

Operations

Obviously, such a situation should be completely avoided in the first place. The best way to do this is to run excellent operations.

This includes a test call with the patient by the telehealth coordinator before their first ever video consultation to just make sure there are no technical problems at the patient end. Better still, the video consultation software should allow for the patient to make an automated test call into a virtual telehealth coordinator. This is excellency in operations.

If the workflow from booking to holding a video consultation is as automated as possible and hardly ever is it necessary to include a human into the process, that's excellency in operations.

If the computer systems involved in supporting the workflow are always available and 100% reliable, that's excellency in operations.

Automation

Working hard at automating processes, making them scalable and reliable is the basis for a scalable and sustainable digital service offering.

QUICK EXERCISE

What issues in your process do you need to consider that are likely to cause service disruptions? Do they have to do with human failure or computer system failure? What can you do to minimise such incidents?

46

EMBRACE NEW CHARGING MODELS, WITH AND WITHOUT MEDICARE

Making an income

One of the key challenges of making a video consultation service sustainable is the financial side of things: how are you going to charge patients for it.

Medicare

In Australia, most healthcare businesses are concerned about reimbursements by Medicare. There are a couple of video consultation services that can currently be reimbursed by Medicare, all of which focus on bringing more access to rural and remote areas. To take advantage of these services, a patient has to seek healthcare access in a defined area, the so-called "telehealth eligible area" of Australia.

The key current reimbursement models for telehealth are:

- The so-called "dual care" arrangement where a rural patient sits with their local GP and receives a specialist consultation via video. Both the specialist and the GP's fee are covered by Medicare – though there may be a gap payment for the patient. In this model, the GP clinic works like a reliable and tested hub that the specialist can make repeat appointments with. Note that it doesn't have to be a GP, but it can also be a nurse, aboriginal health worker, nurse practitioner, other specialist or midwife that is at the rural end with the patient. This model also applies to a optometrist – ophthalmologist dual care consultation.
- The "Better Access" scheme, where 7 out of 10 mental health services direct to patient can be provided and reimbursed via Medicare per patient per calendar year. The services may be GP-focused psychological strategies services, psychological therapy services, or Allied Health focused psychological strategies.
- The "Better Access" scheme also applies to 7 out of 10 mental health group therapy services.
- Case conferences of multidisciplinary teams to establish and coordinate the management of the care needs of the patient.

- Professional attendances provided to a patient individually or in a group under the new Health Care Homes model.

You might be surprised about how many reimbursement models already exist for rural and remote consultations. It's worth checking the MBS Online system for your clinicians' specialties. There are new initiatives appearing as well, so keep a look out at the changes that Medicare introduces in the telehealth space. You can also contact your professional association to find out more and lobby them to encourage Medicare to embrace online consultations as equally effective to in-person consultations. Plenty of research exists to support this argument.

Note that outside of the Medicare environment, video conferencing is already widespread practice in State public health systems.

Gap

Many healthcare consultations require private payment of a gap and most Allied Health consultations that a patient seeks cannot be reimbursed by Medicare in Australia at all. There is a simple model that a video consultation service in these areas can follow: simply charge the patient as much for a video consultation as they would pay for an in-person consultation. Add a small telehealth fee if you like but be aware that telehealth can also save you money, e.g. if clinicians can provide consultations from home outside of office hours.

By calling out that the consultation will cost the patient as much as an in-person fee, the patient realises that they are not getting taken advantage of. By calling out the telehealth fee, the patient gets to value the convenience factor: their travel time, travel expenses, potential waiting time and any other inconveniences created by interrupting a routine day with a clinician visit.

Private Health Insurance

About 50% of the Australian population has private health cover. Interestingly, private health insurers have taken a different route to telehealth than Medicare: rather than describing what types of video consultations they cover and pay for, several insurers have decided to purchase or partner with video consultation services and offer those services at a discount. For example, HCF have partnered with GP2U to offer online GP services at a 20% discount. General rebates for video consultations are not yet available. However, in 2018 as I'm writing this book, the interest of private healthcare insurers in video consultations is increasing and they have started conversations with different professional associations to discuss their concerns and come to a better understanding.

Corporate Health

Organisations in Australia have to be insured for workers compensation. Every work injury that occurs costs a company lots of money in lost work time as well as increased premiums, even if it is just a slip on wet stairs. One of our customers had a clever idea: they are offering a video consultation program to corporates that will result in less workers compensation claims by offering free physiotherapy sessions on the job to workers. This reduces the injury rate substantially and has many positive results in the corporate workforce, making it worthwhile for the employer to fund such a program.

This shows that if you think outside the box that is put around healthcare with Medicare and private health insurance, you might find some opportunities in your market that are untapped for video consultations.

Not-government-organisations (NGOs)

Another great use of video consultations is by NGOs and not-for-profit organisations that deliver support for targeted community groups of patients, such as for rare diseases. There is insight in such organisations that the public health system has often yet to embrace and these organisations are able to provide services to their members that can help them cope better with their illnesses in a more holistic manner. Video consultations by Allied Health practitioners are often part of what is being provided as a service, funded through donations and provided affordably to patients.

QUICK EXERCISE

Think outside the box about who you might be able to partner with to grow your video consultation access to patients. Who needs your practice's capabilities the most, but may not yet be reached? Who can you partner with to get funding?

47

STACKING UP CHANGE PROJECTS - KAIZEN

Successive change

We've previously talked about the need to not just run a single project, but to consider digital transformation as a sequence of projects that each make a small change to your healthcare business, ultimately bringing about the large goal that you've imagined at the beginning of this book.

Kaizen

We've mentioned this philosophy before but want to dig a bit more into the details here. Kaizen is a Japanese word that means "change for better" and supports a process of constant, continuous improvement through small changes.

The philosophy first appeared when several Japanese businesses, shortly after World War II, embraced the idea that doing things the way they have always been done was a bad idea, especially when better options were available that would make them more competitive. Inspired by western competitors and manufacturing methods, "Kaizen" came to be synonymous with company-wide efforts to improve upon and intelligently streamlined business practices and manufacturing methods while simultaneously respecting the product, craft, or the people involved with making it.

Continuous improvement

This kind of continuous improvement can be broken down into six steps:

1. **Standardise:** come up with a process for a specific activity that's repeatable and organised.
2. **Measure:** examine whether the process is efficient using quantifiable data, like time to complete, hours spent, etc.
3. **Compare:** compare your measurements against your requirements. Does this process save time? Does it take too much time? Does it accomplish the desired result?

4. **Innovate:** search for new, better ways to do the same work or achieve the same result. Look for smarter, more efficient routes to the same end-goal that boost productivity.

5. **Standardise:** create repeatable, defined processes for those new, more efficient activities.

6. **Repeat:** go back to step one and start again.

It may seem exhausting, but once it's part of your mental approach to work, or your company (or team) culture, it will feel very natural. If you're always looking for better ways to do things, and you're always willing to give them a try, it's just a step up to formalise it and make sure everyone's on the same page.

Embracing technology

The best way to go about creating new services – and embracing technology – is to come up with a small step for a specific activity that can improve productivity of the business. In the case of video consultations, it may be that a single function in your business is taken online, such as the reporting of test results from a pathology test, or a weekly check-in for therapy-based businesses. That makes patients, clinicians and staff acquainted with video consultations. Then increasingly complex services can be taken online over time

---

QUICK EXERCISE

Reconsider what series of improvements/new services you could focus your launch of video consultation services. Did you pick the smallest possible change? Try not to look too far ahead so you can be flexible with the results.

48

OPPORTUNITIES FOR GROWTH

Business as usual

You have a successful model for video consultations when your business starts running smoothly with them, your existing patients start increasingly embracing it, and you start attracting new patients through word of mouth or one of your marketing exercises. Now is the time to start thinking even bigger.

Opportunity for growth

Is it a particular service that you are starting to get known for? Does it make sense to hire more people to offer this particular service? Would it be possible to hire people that work from home?

Remote workforce

Often there are very qualified people in your domain, but they have family or location restrictions and can therefore not work for the best employer in their field. Video consultations offer a completely new flexibility in hiring such people. It's not without its challenges though – you have to try much harder to make them part of your organisation's culture and events. There are many ways in which a remote workforce can interact with a local one. For example, make sure to hold all-hands meetings over video conference so they can participate. Make sure to regularly catch up with them one-on-one over video conference to ask how their past week was, whether there are any issues and what you could do to improve things. Make sure they also communicate frequently with their peers and not just with patients.

Subsidiaries

Another opportunity for growth is that you can now offer services nation-wide and open subsidiaries of your practice that follow a similar model to yours. Since the services offered in the subsidiaries will be standardised on the model you are offering in your practice, suddenly you can balance the patients across these two practices. This can apply even to walk-in patients – if they don't mind who they are seeing, you can offer them a patient booth to talk with one of your remote clinicians. It's another means of transforming your in-person customers into video consultation customers.

International reach

Once you've reached national borders, what stops you from offering your services internationally? Well, yes, you have to make sure you are insured and licensed to offer your services in other countries. But from a patient viewpoint, they are just after the best service provider. If that's you, they don't really care where you are. You might start with offering such an international service to your local patients while they are travelling. But later you can also offer it to expats or overseas patients that speak your language or bring a translator along.

QUICK EXERCISE

Every large opportunity starts small. If you are just starting out on your digital health journey, don't worry too much about how to scale it yet. But eventually, when your video consultations are successful, you will be able to extend your model beyond the boundaries of your local practice. Where do you want to take it tomorrow?

CHECKLIST: IS YOUR PROJECT EXECUTED SUCCESSFULLY?

Consider what a successful, sustainable and scalable video consultation service looks like for you:

1. Are your staff and clinicians treating video consultations as just another service?
2. Are your patients booking video consultations regularly and telling others about it?
3. Do you have many success stories to tell?
4. Are you routinely running marketing exercises around video consultations?
5. Are you ready to scale up your business model to other locations and to clinicians working from home?
6. Have you found a specialty that makes you stand out from other clinics with video consultations?
7. Are you known across the country by clinicians for the specific service you are providing?
8. Could you offer it to anybody on the planet?

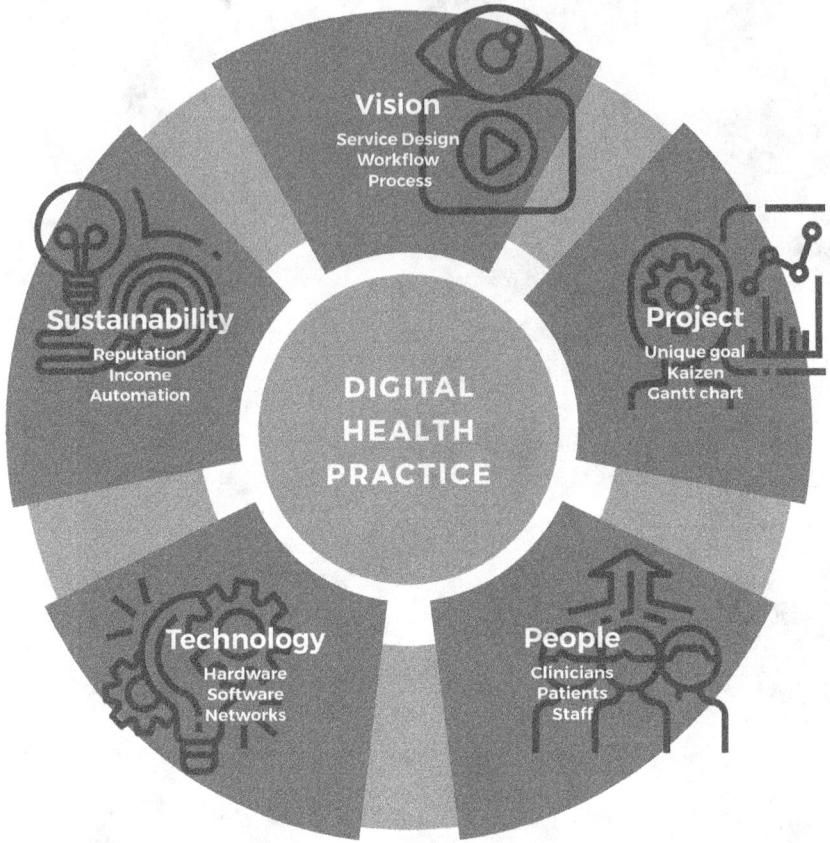

Vision
Service Design
Workflow
Process

Project
Unique goal
Kaizen
Gantt chart

Sustainability
Reputation
Income
Automation

DIGITAL
HEALTH
PRACTICE

Technology
Hardware
Software
Networks

People
Clinicians
Patients
Staff

The purpose of this book was to provide you, the healthcare professional, with ideas for transforming your business for a digital future.

We've walked you through the different steps necessary in setting up a successful, sustainable video consultation service. All the way from building your vision of the service, through creating a transformation project, getting the key people on board, getting the technology right, to making the service business-as-usual.

Keep in mind that you don't have to do it right the first time. The case studies that we showed are from people who tweaked their service a lot before getting it just right. And they will continue to tweak it as they continue to scale it. So, get started with something small – even if it's just a single practitioner – and grow from there.

A couple of key things to get right at the beginning are to pick a single service to get started with, target specific patients and clinicians, get your practice personnel on board, pick a good technology partner and think about how you will make money from the service. When you succeed, you will have created more flexibility for your patients and clinicians but also made more money along the way and transformed your business sustainably.

It will not always be a simple journey, but don't give up. Find some support from others that have been down the same path – maybe through your industry association, through conferences, or even in an online forum such as a Facebook group or Google community, or one of the clinician networks, e.g. Somo or the Mayo Clinic Social Media Network.

What's the next step you are going to take?

I'd love to hear about your challenges and solutions – feel free to contact me at **silvia@coviu.com** .

REFERENCES

These are telehealth books that were used as background reading for this book and are recommended for their specific areas of focus.

Cuyler R. & Holland D. *Implementing Telemedicine: Completing Projects On Target On Time On Budget*, 2012.

A comprehensive book for the introduction of major telehealth projects in *hospitals* with lots of focus on project planning, budgeting and outcome metrics. This can be a bit overkill for primary healthcare projects.

Eren H. & Webster J.G. *Telehealth and Mobile Health*, 2016.

This book has a large focus on robots, *telesurgery* and telenursing, in case you are after modern hospital applications of telehealth.

Jones C. *Webcam Savvy for Telemedicine*, 2017.

A very practical book for all clinicians that are a bit camera-shy and need to build some confidence around *camera skills*.

Jones L.D. *The Truth about Telehealth: Why A Revolutionary Industry Has Failed To Deliver And How It Can Still Be A Game-Changer For Healthcare*, 2018.

A US-centric book about how telehealth in the US is broken because *employee benefits brokers*, insurance companies and major telehealth companies are not ultimately interested in a huge uptake and don't market these solutions sufficiently.

Kamenca, A. *Telemedicine: A Practical Guide for Professionals*, 2017.

A comprehensive book about the operational, legal, financial, clinical, and technology elements needed to develop successful telemedicine programs in the US. It has a keen focus on developing a *business case*.

Krohn R., Metcalf D. & Salber P. *Connected Health: Improving Care, Safety, and Efficiency with Wearables and IoT Solution*, 2017.

This book conducts a focused examination of *wearables* and the IoT space as an explosive niche of the Connect Health market. There is lots of strategic information about devices and their impact but little on how to introduce them successfully into your organisation.

Lyuboslavky V. *Telemedicine and Telehealth 2.0: A Practical Guide for Medical Providers and Patients*, **2015.**

Like many of the earlier books on telehealth, this one provides an overview of different types of telehealth *technologies* and how to solve your hardware, software and network setup. There is no focus on process changes and business challenges.

Oldenburg J. (ed) *Participatory Healthcare: A Person-Centered Approach to Healthcare Transformation*, **2016.**

This book is written through the lens of *patients*, caregivers, healthcare representatives and families, highlighting new models of interaction between providers and patients and what people would like in their healthcare experience.

Schulder Rheuban K. & Krupinski E.A. *Understanding Telehealth*, **2018.**

A book that goes through a lot of the *common use cases of modern telehealth*: telestroke, obstetrics, teleophthalmology, critical care, teledermatology, telepsychiatry, remote patient monitoring, paediatrics, etc. Very good to understand potential projects.

Yellowlees P. & Shore J.H. *Telepsychiatry and Health Technologies – A Guie for Mental Health Professionals*, **2018.**

An in-depth book for *psychiatrists and other mental health care professionals* about the challenges encountered in the information age and how to leverage them in practice with patients. It has a US focus particularly with respect to reimbursement opportunities and the legal and regulatory environment. The US is the most developed country in adopting telepsychiatry, so there is much to learn from the experience of the 32 individuals who contributed to the book.

INDEX

S

scientific literature 56

service design 29

Skype 16, 20, 29, 43, 54, 71, 109, 134

software 15, 16, 28, 29, 30, 33, 34, 35, 36, 37, 38, 39, 41, 54, 56, 61, 71, 79, 82, 85, 101, 102, 109, 110, 111, 112, 113, 114, 115, 119, 125, 126, 127, 128, 129, 131, 132, 133, 134, 135, 137, 138, 143, 144, 145, 147, 148, 159, 160

solution provider 15, 56, 82, 83

specialists 21, 25, 43, 44, 97, 98

speech pathology 15, 32, 42, 43, 75, 133, 157

stay-at-work rate 41

suitability 33

support 26, 29, 30, 40, 42, 43, 44, 63, 72, 75, 78, 82, 87, 97, 101, 105, 109, 110, 111, 114, 125, 131, 132, 133, 134, 135, 136, 147, 148, 159, 162, 163, 171

sustainability 31, 38, 39, 61, 79, 150, 155

T

telehealth 15, 21, 23, 24, 26, 27, 29, 32, 38, 41, 44, 56, 63, 64, 70, 75, 82, 90, 91, 93, 101, 102, 106, 107, 110, 111, 112, 114, 115, 116, 117, 120, 121, 128, 135, 136, 139, 159, 161, 162, 172

telehealth coordinator 44, 63, 75, 82, 93, 101, 106, 107, 110, 111, 112, 114, 115, 116, 117, 128, 135, 159, 160

telemedicine 23, 24, 136

telepractice 16, 32, 42

test call 33, 112, 113, 116, 159

therapy 21, 24, 32, 49, 51, 58, 75, 86, 98, 132, 161, 165

training 15, 26, 29, 41, 42, 75, 83, 100, 101, 105, 111, 112, 113, 114, 116, 121, 134

transformation 30, 68

V

value-based care 21

video consultations 15, 16, 17, 20, 22, 23, 24, 25, 26, 27, 28, 29, 30, 32, 33, 34, 35, 36, 38, 39, 41, 43, 44, 45, 49, 50, 52, 53, 54, 58, 59, 60, 63, 64, 65, 66, 69, 70, 74, 75, 76, 78, 81, 82, 83, 84, 86, 87, 88, 89, 90, 91, 92, 93, 97, 98, 99, 101, 102, 103, 106, 107, 109, 110, 111, 112, 113, 114, 115, 116, 119, 121, 125, 126, 127, 128, 129, 130, 131, 132, 133, 134, 135, 136, 137, 138, 139, 140, 141, 142, 143, 144, 145, 148, 152, 153, 154, 155, 157, 159, 160, 161, 162, 163, 165, 166, 167, 168, 171

vision 30, 36, 40, 43, 48, 49, 50, 53, 54, 55, 56, 57, 60, 61, 62, 66, 69, 79, 97, 106, 108, 134, 171

W

waiting room 44, 126, 132

waiting rooms 54, 135

website 30, 44, 74, 75, 118, 119, 120

workflow 15, 28, 29, 31, 37, 50, 54, 57, 59, 60, 63, 64, 66, 69, 72, 105, 107, 110, 113, 114, 125, 126, 132, 133, 134, 137, 139, 140, 145, 146, 147, 148, 160

ABOUT THE AUTHOR

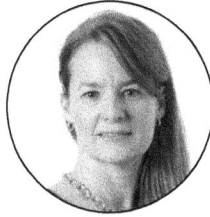

Silvia Pfeiffer's background is in Computer Science, but she has always harboured a passion for healthcare. In fact, when finishing school, she intended to study medicine, but an attendance of a small operation on her father at the local doctor made it clear she wasn't cut out for it. So she turned to computers and is now coming back full circle to help practitioners and healthcare businesses embrace digital developments in healthcare and to improve access to healthcare for the many patients that are disadvantaged by location, physique or mentality from getting the best help.

Silvia's story is also one of several continents. In May 1999, after finishing her PhD in Computer Science in Germany, Silvia moved her family and herself to Australia to follow an invitation by the Australian government research organisation CSIRO (Commonwealth Scientific Research Organisation). She was to work as a post-doc continuing her research on audio/video content analysis – what would later be known as video recognition, a field of artificial intelligence.

Her first focus was on analysing and automatically transcribing spoken words in videos with a goal to automating subtitling and captioning and helping deaf people get better access to video content. In 1999, that was quite an audacious goal, because speech recognition quality was pretty atrocious. YouTube's auto-caption functionality is only accurate enough to be usable since about 2017. The CSIRO project in 2000 proved that automated tools could speed up the work of a captioner and now, 18 years later, we can mostly automate caption creation – with some additional human Q&A.

Soon afterwards, as Silvia was exploring increasingly more ways of automatically extracting interesting information from videos, she started considering how that might influence the future of our human relationship with video. This was back in the days when

Adobe Flash started to become the default standard for publishing videos on the Web and the videos we were watching were stamp-sized. Silvia predicted that within just a couple of years we would see the number of videos published on the Web to increase exponentially and somebody would need to figure out how to crawl, index, and search these videos.

Silvia set herself the task of making video a prime citizen on the Web: something that Web search engines could analyse and understand, that users could easily find and interact with. In 2000, she invented "Annodex" – annotated and indexed video files for the Web. By 2006, as her predictions started coming true, the W3C – the World Wide Web Consortium – the standards body that defines all formats for the Web – started addressing the challenges of video on the Web and Silvia contributed.

It was the year YouTube was created and Silvia created her first start-up – a company called Vquence that was to provide a video search engine and a new, efficient experience for video consumption. Vquence lasted 10 years but didn't end up becoming the large consumer platform Silvia originally envisaged.

By 2010, video had indeed become ubiquitous on the Web and new platforms such as Netflix started springing up and Silvia worked for Mozilla, then Google on improving video on the Web. The next challenge was to bring video conferencing to the Web browser to make video calls more ubiquitous.

Video conferencing was a completely different challenge to anything the Web had faced before, because the paradigm of the Web had to change from being a mere video-content consumption platform to a live interaction platform between users that were connecting from different Web browsers. This is called a peer-to-peer use case and didn't sit well with the traditional client-server architecture of the Web.

As Google decided to take on the challenge and bring it to the W3C, a new project sprang to life and was called WebRTC – real-time communications for the Web. Silvia joined the new working group and wrote and published one of the first demonstrators of having WebRTC work in a Google Chrome Web browser in 2012.

In 2013, Silvia returned to NICTA/CSIRO to apply WebRTC to healthcare. In the *SWAY* project at the Royal Far West School in Manly, speech pathologists were providing speech therapy services to students in rural and remote NSW schools. Their existing tools were completely inadequate to work with children. Silvia programmed a modern solution that was used for three years before being replaced by Coviu.

Coviu is the platform Silvia's team built in CSIRO. It was spun out into a stand-alone company with venture capital investment in 2018. Coviu provides a modern integrated telehealth solution to care providers. Many Allied Health, GP and specialist practices have signed on to serve their own patients via video consultations on Coviu. Silvia and her team have learnt a lot about what works and what doesn't when setting up a new video consultation service, and Silvia's goal is to share these learnings through this book.